Part I

Electro-acupuncture Primer

on Electro-acupuncture
acc. to Reinhold Voll, M.D.

compiled by
Fritz Werner, M. Sc.

Part II

Interpretation of the Rules of the Energy Exchange in Acupuncture
and

Part III

Choice of the Examination Place in Electro-acupuncture acc. to Voll (EAV)
by Reinhold Voll, M.D.

Translated by Hartwig Schuldt, M.D., M.Sc.

4th German edition 1978
1st English edition 1979

Medizinisch Literarische Verlagsgesellschaft mbH · Uelzen

Contents

Appendix

Part II

Interpretation of the acupuncture rules and energy exchanges

Part III
Choice of the examination place in Electro-acupuncture acc. to Voll

Preface

The teachings of electro-acupuncture acc. to *Voll* form part of modern medicine after developing over recent years. The results of investigations and experiences in electro-acupuncture diagnosis and therapy as well as medication-testing are reflected by many publications. I hope that this booklet will serve as an introduction to the practical and technical management of electro-acupuncture thus closing a still existing gap. This primer of electro-acupuncture has been compiled in a fashion that questions are being asked and answered subsequently.

It has not been possible each time to seperate questions related to technology from those of biology and medicine. Therefore, this booklet has been controlled by Dr. *Voll*. It does not claim perfection to replace the thorough training in courses, but should help to memorize the subject more easily.

The teachings of electro-acupuncture acc. to *Voll* have developed rapidly. New results have been found and published in ample literature. In English excist five books and one supplement. This is the 6th book.

Also, the electro-acupuncture apparatuses have been advanced. The vacuum tubes in the old instruments were replaced by modern transistors and by pressed cards of connections (chips). The multiple experiences in using the apparatuses have been evaluated: thus the four-quadrant diagnosis and -therapy were incorporated into the apparatuses.

The curve forms of the therapy currents were added by the utilization and introduction of the "negative saw tooth" (the direct current negative relaxation oscillation). The outer dimensions of the instruments were reduced as well as their weight.

Basically, the construction and performance of the instruments remained unchanged rendering all the results achieved by the employed electro-acupuncture instruments acc. to *Voll* comparable, even to-day.

This booklet contains many repititions as it is meant to serve as a manual.

Stuttgart, June 1979 *Dr. F. Werner*

To the reader of this electro-acupuncture primer

Dr. *Werner* has participated in more than 100 introductory courses on electro-acupuncture lasting two days each. He has helped me with technical problems. Furthermore, he has given a talk on the technical foundations of the electro-acupuncture instruments acc. to Voll as well as on the make-up of the examination place for carrying out electro-acupuncture.

As a manufacturer and agent of the instruments he has, in addition, answered many questions raised by the participants of courses, which could not be answered in the courses themselves. Many questions were asked repeatedly. Therefore, Dr. *Werner* has compiled a great deal of these questions in the form of questions and answers in this electro-acupuncture primer. Dr. *Werner* can master the subject of electro-acupuncture having participated in the development of electro-acupuncture diagnosis and therapy from the start. As to the medical questions in the electro-acupuncture primer, I have assisted Dr. *Werner* when necessary.

I thank the ML-Publisher, who has edited the entire literature on electro-acupuncture acc. to Voll, for printing this electro-acupuncture primer.

In the second part of this booklet I have, for the first time, written down my outlines in the course-work on the interpretation of the rules of the energy exchange as diagnostic hints for preventive therapy and for the therapy of organ diseases, since comprehensive literature up to now is missing on that.

I believe to have enriched Dr. *Werners* enlarged and revised electro-acupuncture primer.

November 1974   *Dr. R. Voll*

Preface

The fact that it was necessary after four years to print a new edition of the Electro-Acupuncture Primer is sufficient proof, that make-up and style of this rather complicated matter has been generally acclaimed by the readers. The contents of this booklet has been revised and brought up to latest standards.

Dr. *Voll* deserves a *thank-you* for checking the manuscript. Likewise, I want to extend a *thank-you* to the ML-Publisher in Uelzen for printing this primer.

Last not least, I wish to thank Dr. *Schuldt* for preparing this excellent translation together with some corrections.

Stuttgart, February 1978   *Dr. F. Werner*

Preface

In the enlarged 4th edition I have enlarged the interpretation of the maximum times in classical acupuncture for diagnostic hints as to organ diseases by considering the beginning of complaints in four further symptoms, i.e., vomiting, fits of asthma, eruptions of sweat and fits of dizziness. This is supported by the corresponding case reports.

For preventive therapy I have shown the rule of the crossed relations between left and right pulse loci together with corresponding pathophysiologic explanations.

In carrying out preventive therapy this rule was exemplified by a heart disease to show the better numerical results of therapy.

The English edition of this book also includes a work published in 1978 by me on "The choice of the examination place in electro-acupuncture acc. to Voll (EAV)". This paper is very important for the beginner in order to avoid faulty readings in patients caused by different kinds of electrical fields, which may influence the patient adversely, or by electro-statically charged synthetic materials. The ideal pre-requisites for the examination room in EAV are described in the final chapter.

Plochingen, June 1979 *Dr. R. Voll*

The arrangement of an electro-acupuncture examination place.

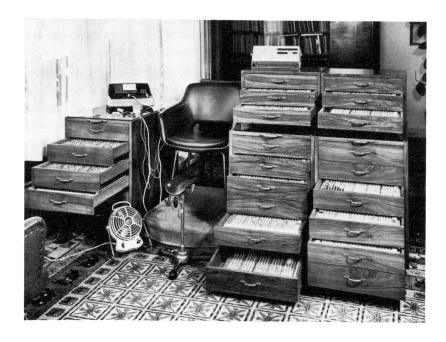

Description of the examination place

Consisting of:

1. At least two, but usually several sliding cases to accommodate the medications. Material: Wood!

   Sliding cases for accommodating drawings are offered among office furniture. These sliding cases are also useful for the placing of medication boards or residual medications in their original boxes. Such cases are made out of metal (iron or steel).

   Cases resting on well insulating floors (plastic material flooring) should not be charged by static electricity (by touching charged objects or persons). They should, therefore, be properly grounded. Your electrician may give useful advice on that.

2. An elevated platform consisting of wood, preferably also a wooden chair (without artificial material lining) for the patients.

3. An adjustable footrest.

4. An EAV-apparatus according to your choice including the necessary accessories.

5. A fan for warm or cool air.

6. A sufficient number of medication boards in the cases (measuring 45 cm broad, 53 cm long, 4,5 cm thick. Weight: no more than 4 kg).

7. Bowls containing cotton tissue both dry and moist.

1.

1. Description of the electro-acupuncture apparatuses according to Voll (EAV-apparatuses)

1.1 Production and sales of the apparatuses:

1.1.1. Kraiss und Fritz, Neckarstr. 182, D-7000 Stuttgart 1, Telephone (0711) 28 32 21

1.1.2. Pitterling-Electronic, Akademiestr. 5, D-8000 München 40, Telephone (089) 34 72 81

1.2. The various EAV-models

1.2.1. *K+F-Diatherapuncteur,* transistorized, net supplied. These apparatuses are still in use (some of them for more than fifteen years) but are no longer manufactured.

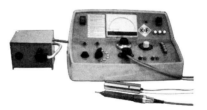

Diatherapuncteur 1.2.1.

1.2.2. *Dermatron,* transistorized, containing a rechargeable battery.

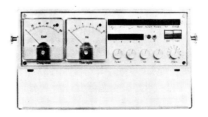

Dermatron 1.2.2.

1.

1.2.3. *EAV-Portable,* operated on dry batteries.

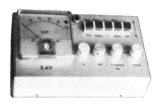

EAV-Kleingerät 1.2.3

To 1.2.1 (Showing the development of EAV-apparatuses).

Some outlines on the *K+F-Diatherapuncteur* shall be given as to the utilization of this apparatus in practice. The basic make-up of this instrument had been leading the way for all later modern technical equipment in EAV.

1.2.1. a)

The name of the *K+F-Diatherapuncteur* implies that the apparatus is made by the **K**raiss & **F**riz company in Stuttgart, Neckarstr. 182. It had been devised as a combined diagnostic and therapeutic apparatus using as a working hypothesis the old teachings of classical acupuncture from China. The term of *EAV* had been suggested by Dr. *Kramer,* Nürnberg, for ,,**E**lectro-**A**cupuncture according to **V**oll''.

1.2.1. b) (Only for the older apparatuses)

The apparatus is connected to the mains (socket) of 220 volt, alternating current, and 50 Hertz. When the mains contain different voltages, these have to be transformed to a voltage of 220 volt. Transformer output approx. 100 VA. (volt times ampères).

The apparatus contains a device for the constancy of voltage plus/minus 10 per cent of the basic voltage. A fuse in the apparatus is for 0,5 amp. To assure the grounding of the casing of the *K+F-Diatherapuncteur* in practical use, only contacts with grounding should be made (protection grounding sockets).

When however, in exceptional cases such as near the bedside, there are no protection grounding sockets available, the apparatus may be used as well yet yielding normal functions.

1.2.1. c)

Those apparatuses manufactured before 1974 and sooner have a separate unit for the transformer and the fuse (see Fig. 1.2.1.). The connection cords (leads) to the apparatus are only meant for low voltage (20 volt).

1.2.1. d)

The apparatuses under c) are fully transistorized, facilitating also quadrant derivations, negative direct current relaxation oscillations (kipp) as well as acoustic pointfinding.

1.2.1. e)

To facilitate a more practical utilization of the apparatuses, the four most important functions have been programmed for the use of dials, these being:

1. Diagnosis and therapy by hand (by means of a stylus) using automatic frequency changes from 0.8 to 10.0 Hertz (by depressing the knob on the stylus).
2. Diagnosis and therapy by hand (like under 1) using specific frequency (by depressing the knob on the stylus).
3. Permanent therapy using specific and (stepless by gradable) sliding frequencies. The frequency may be tuned by means of

1.

the middle handwheel and the corresponding scaling for a ten-spiral potentiometer.

4. Permanent therapy using an automatic switch to shift from diagnosis (approx. 3 sec.) to therapy (approx. 10 sec.) and vice versa as well as specific frequency (to be tuned from 0.8 to 10.0 Hertz).

5. Permanent therapy using automatic frequency changes (from 0.8 to 10.0 Hertz approx. each 3 min.)= wave swing (sweep).

6. Permanent therapy using automatic frequency changes (see under 5) in addition to automatic changing from diagnosis to therapy and vice versa = wave swing plus diagnostic control.

1.2.1. f)

The diagnosis part of the *K+F-Diatherapuncteur* consists of an ohmicmeter, in other words, of a resistance measurement device with a high internal resistance of approx. 1 megohm. In order to avoid, that the polarisation tension of the skin, arising between the metal of the electrode and the sweat of the skin disturbs the measurement, a considerable zero-point displacement has been provided with the apparatus responding only to a contact resistance of approx. 600 kiloohms. Every part for diagnosis is calibrated by means of a phantom, thus making possible the comparison between readings taken by different apparatuses. Readings taken from the body are based on "technical direct current" showing an undulation of less than 0.1 per cent. Older apparatuses sometimes have a slightly higher undulation. (Remark: The term of undulation refers to the superimposition of an alternating current on top of a direct current.) However, this undulation plays no major roll in diagnostics, after it turned out that other apparatuses using alternating current for measurements (such as those used by *W. Schmidt,* München), yield equal results with respect to the indicator drop, consuming, however, much more time in comparison to EAV-apparatuses operated on direct current. In the scale's mid-position of the instrument ($=50$), there is a voltage of approx. 1 volt between the two electrodes. A current of approx. 9 mikroamp. (9×10^{-6} amp.) is then passing through the body to be measured. (See also page 88 for the calibration curve of the diagnostic instrument.)

1.2.1. g)

As to the therapeutic part of the *K+F-Diatherapuncteur,* the frequency used (oscillations per sec.) may be adjusted both by hand or automatically, ranging between 0.8 to 10.0 Hertz, in addition to changing the intensity of alternating relaxation oscillations between 0.0 and approx. 400 volt (see also under e). 400 volt refers to the peak-to-peak voltage obtainable between the positive and the negative peaks of the curve. This can only be verified by means of an oscilloscope or any corresponding measurement device, but not by means of a customary voltmeter.

Forms of current output:

Alternating relaxation oscillations = impulse = charging (increasing);

positive direct current relaxation oscillations = positive sawtooth = discharging (decreasing);

negative direct current relaxation oscillations = negative sawtooth = pseudo-charging (increasing).

These individual current characteristics may be chosen by depressing the corresponding knob as indicated on the apparatus. (See appendix: Therapeutic currents applied on the acupuncture point on page 104 and 105 ff).

1.2.1. h)

The normal electrode output of the apparatus is usually switched on diagnosis. When the knob on the stylus is depressed or when "permanent therapy" is turned on, a green lamp is shining up indicating that the electrodes are connected to the therapeutic part of the instrument. In the Dermatron apparatus a small lamp in the upper right part of the corresponding measurement scale indicates that either diagnosis or therapy (frequency measurements) is turned on.

1.2.1. i)

The electrodes are connected to the instrument by means of a shielded cord (lead) using an unmistakable six-prong contact. The stylus is connected by means of a powerless tripleprong contact.

1.

Note the groove and tongue. The point-electrode is mounted on top of the stylus by means of a screw-thread (positive pole).

The hand-electrode has to be connected to the black or blue banana plug of the diagnosis cord (lead)= minus pole.

1.2.1. k)

The four quadrants of the body may be derived for diagnosis and therapy by means of the denoted sockets (HH = hand-hand and FF = foot-foot.

red socket:	hand right
black socket:	hand left
green socket:	foot right
yellow socket:	foot left

The pressbuttons on the right side of the instrument facilitate the equally polarized connections:

HH	=	hand - hand
LS	=	left hand - left foot (left side)
RS	=	right hand - right foot (right side)
FF	=	foot - foot.

For further outlines on conductance measurements, see 9.5 and 14.2.2.

To 1.2.2.

1.2.2. a)

The *Dermatron* apparatus made by Pitterling-Electronic, D-8000 München 40, Akademiestr. 5, is a further development of the *K+F-Diatherapuncteur* and of the electro-acupuncture devices according to *Voll.*

It is characterized by:

a) low weight
b) compact design
c) rechargeable accumulator.

1.2.2. b)

The functions achieved by the *Dermatron* apparatus correspond exactly to those of the *K+F-Diatherapuncteur*. They are comparable among all existing EAV-instruments (Electro-acupuncture-instruments according to *Voll*).

Individual performances:

Diagnosis = D
Therapy = T
Wave swing = WS
specific frequency = Hand + Freq.
automatic output = Autom.

charging =
discharging =
pseudocharging =
acoustic point finding = sound
quadrant derivation = I, II, III, IV
intensity

are clearly marked and symbolized. The frequency may be turned on and read both specifically and by means of the wave swing (sweep) using a measurement scale denoted "Hz" (Hertz). When diagnosis (D) is turned on the toggle switch next to the main switch a lamp shines up in the right upper corner of the diagnosis instrument.

When therapy (T) is turned on, a lamp shines up in the right upper corner of the scale for therapy frequency. The Dermatron apparatus should be recharged constantly from the mains when it is in permanent use; but in its actual application, it may be separated from the mains. When the instrument is out of use for a longer period of time, it should be recharged at least every four weeks for 12 hours.

1.

The Dermatron apparatus may be connected to a recorder. The calibration of the diagnostic indicator is done by the two dials denoted "0" and "100". For point finding, use the point finding cord (lead), depress the key *point* and use the dial *point* (see No. 21.2 last paragraph).

To 1.2.3.

1.2.3. a)
The *EAV-Portable* is used both for diagnosis and therapy in electro-acupuncture:
– no connection to the mains
– easy to transport
– to be used in electro-acupuncture for decreasing (discharging) and pseudo-increasing (pseudo-charging) as well as medication testing.

1.2.3. b)

Its voltage is supplied by three mono batteries (such as Varta Super Dry 282, mono 1,5 V IEC R 20).

1.2.3. c)
The output functions of the instrument correspond to the large instruments. A wave swing is also provided. The curve characteristics for therapy are restricted to the positive decreasing and the negative pseudo-increasing sawtooth characteristics only.

These two curve characteristics are considered sufficient to keep pre-treated patients or the medical doctor himself in energetic balance.

In pronounced energetic low voltage, the application of the negative sawtooth, however, will have no lasting effect.

1.2.3. d)
The advantages of the *EAV-Portable* may be summarized as follows:
– light and handy
– dry battery operated

– particularly useful for the family doctor and for traveling
– incorporating a diagnostic and a therapeutic part
– including wave swing and frequency dialing
– two current output characteristics.

2.

2. What is electro-acupuncture all about?

2.1.

Electro-acupuncture is a comprehensive term for all procedures based on measurements or therapy derived from Chinese acupuncture, using modern electronics.

2.2

The word of "Electro-Acupuncture" was first coined by the French acupuncturist Dr. *Roger de la Fuye* in Paris. He combined an electric device (Diathermopuncteur) with the inserted needle in order to apply on certain points of the skin – the so-called acupuncture points – as an additional therapeutic stimulus a diathermia-current lasting 1/8 to 2 seconds via the inserted needle.

2.2.1.

Acupuncture analgesia, in use since approx. 1970, applies electrical current to inserted needles, and is also referred to as electro-acupuncture.

In contrast, current impulses used in electro-acupuncture according to *Voll* are not appropriate for analgesia.

2.3.

Independent of the above outlines, *Voll* and *Werner,* as early as 1953, developed an instrument for applying electro-acupuncture on the skin without needle pricks. This apparatus was called *"Electropuncteur"* and after the protest of Dr. *de la Fuye* was re-named *K+F-Diatherapuncteur".* The term of electro-acupuncture today is so widespread that a special definition has to be given, for which this booklet should render sufficient help.

2.4.

Preliminary tests for this apparatus were started in 1953 based on hints given to Dr. *Werner* for the production of an instrument capable of objectively locating acupuncture points. Dr. *Voll* took over these hints and formulated the following conditions:

1. After the location of the points they should be rendered measurable.

2. A subsequent electric treatment of the points using low frequency current impulses should be made possible by means of impulse characteristics differing for "the gold and the silver effects achieved by needles".

3. In addition, after each current impulse, the new measurement value of the acupuncture point should re-establish itself in order to avoid over- or under-treatment.

These conditions established by *Voll* gave rise to the construction und scope of the instrument which was finished in 1955 and then presented to the medical public.

3.

3. What is classical acupuncture?

3.1.

Classical acupuncture has been in use for several thousand years and has been developed by East-Asian peoples based on empirical findings. It has been developed to a stage where one could stimulate certain skin areas of least dimensions – that is, the acupuncture points – in order to achieve organ effects in the body.

3.2

The stimulation of the organs in classical acupuncture is achieved by pricking needles made out of gold, silver, steel, or bamboo on the so-called acupuncture points. The acupuncture point is situated on a "meridian" leading to an organ or to a functional system (circulation or triple-warmer = endocrine system). The topographic positions of the various acupuncture points have been fully described by Dr. R. Voll in stating more than 600 measurement points in electro-acupuncture on anatomic figures.

3.3.

The question arises of how East-Asian natural peoples without knowing electronics, were capable of establishing classical ancient acupuncture.

3.3.1.

We know of animals whose spectrum of perception with respect to eyes and ears and smell is far superior to that of men, exceeding the perception of men considerably. An example for this is the capability of cats to see at night. An explanation for this can only be the capability to register light beams in the infra-red realm. It is thus possible to conclude that some of these natural peoples living several thousand years back were capable of registering infra-red light more strongly than we can today.

3.3.2.

Everybody possessing a temperature higher than his surroundings irradiates infra-red into the space (measurement device:

Bolometer according to *Schwamm*). It became likewise known that acupuncture points on the dorsum of the hand (not on the palm) exhibit a very slight depression of the overall surface temperature of the skin. On the basis of this, one may well imagine that natural man in his age could virtually see the relief of irradiated infra-red rays to enable him to pass these findings on to posterity in writing. *Kirlian,* a Russian electronic scientist, first produced this phenomenon in 1939.

3.3.3.

In addition to the above, the *Kirlian* effect should be mentioned with respect to electrophotography.

4.

4. What is understood by a meridian?

4.1.
This is a word which developed in the nomenclature of acupuncture and was likewise taken over by electro-acupuncture according to *Voll*.

4.2.
The meridians are energy pathways formed in the interior organs of the body leading the bio-electric energy to the periphery of the body for its energetic supply.

4.3.
According to ancient acupuncture, there exists a closed energy circulation.

4.4.
The meridians connect the individual acupuncture points. The acupuncture points in turn serve for the interference with the bio-electric energy, thus rendering it measurable.

5.

5. How are measurements in electro-acupuncture carried out on the acupuncture points?

5.1.

The acupuncture points are assumed to be located in the lowest layers of the skin and in the subdermal tissue. Topographically, the acupuncture points are located either on certain osseous situations which may be palpated by the examiner for safe location (mostly situated at the transition zone between the shaft and the capitulum or at the basis of the corresponding bone) or in the muscular tissue, such as when muscular edges intersect. Tentatively, acupuncture points are located at a depth of 2 to 3 mm. Several points are located yet deeper.

For this, refer to: *Voll: Topographic Positions of the Measurement Points in Electro-Acupuncture,* ML-Publisher, Uelzen, 1977, Textual Volume I, Illustrated Volume I and II (anatomic atlases), Textual- and Illustrated Volume III and 1. Supplement to the four volumes on "Topographic positions of the measurement points in Electro-Acupuncture", ML-Publisher, Uelzen, 1978.

5.2.

For measuring an acupuncture point by means of an electrical measurement device, one has to overcome certain magnitudes:

5.2.1.

The resistance of the epidermis including the corium. This resistance may vary considerably depending on age and the present condition of the skin.

5.2.2.

The resistance of the subcutaneous tissue, which is mostly wet rendering the resistance value relatively low or even negligible. The resistance may change in lymphatic stasis around the point itself, indicating that organic insufficiency, related to the corresponding organ, is present.

5.

5.2.3.

The potential of the acupuncture point. In order to measure the potential with greatest accuracy, it is necessary to have the resistances of the corium and the subcutaneous tissue as low as possible.

5.3.

The pressure applied by the stylus and the ball-shaped electrode, the diameter of which is 3 mm, has to reach a value of at least 500 pond (500 gramm) in normally lymphatically drained skin. It may be increased just below reaching a pathologic pressure, that is, a value in which the skin is pierced. According to our experience, this value ranges about 1800 pond (1,8 kg). Within this pressure range, normal skin is compressed to cause an almost constant electrical resistance for the overall reading. This constant value seems to be equal in all individuals thus rendering the individual measurement values comparable at any time. For this, it is most important to hit the acupuncture point when using pressure-constant and registering electrodes, since otherwise faulty measurements would result. There are a number of points, such as on the fingers, whose maximum values best show up when measurements are taken at an angle of 45 degrees (see Illustrated Volume II, Fig. 38 to 41).

5.4.

 In order to carry out a measurement, an instrument is required possessing a very high internal resistance, since the bio-electric energy of the acupuncture point is very small only. Furthermore, the instrument has to yield a current polarized in opposition to the bio-electric energy of the body. The current yielded by the measurement instrument (as a current source) must not exceed the physiologic magnitudes. The connections diagram of the diagnosis instrument of the *K+F-Diatherapuncteur* is shown, in part, on page 86 and the following pages. The transistorized instruments made by *Pitterling-Electronic* also comply with the requirements of electro-acupuncture measurements according to *Voll*.

5.5.

The positive pole of the measurement device is at the stylus, while the negative pole is at the hand-electrode. You may memorize this by considering that the positive pole is the hot pole and what is hot can only be touched when insulated (insulated stylus).

5.6.

The hand-electrode is placed into the patient's hand while the stylus is stroking back and forth across the patient's skin on the acupuncture point. The sensitivity of the measurement device is such that it responds to an external resistance of approx. 600 kiloohms yielding the maximum indicator deviation = 100 in an external resistance of zero = 0.

When one strokes across the skin applying equal pressure, the measurement instrument will show a higher indicator deviation on the acupuncture point. On this point, which yields the higher indicator deviation not yet as the exact measurement reading, you should apply a short maximum pressure with the stylus – the so-called electro-acupuncture pressure – on the measurement point. You will then realize, that the indicator of the measurement device travels upwards becoming stable at a certain value or, alternatively, after reaching the maximum value, starts decreasing more or less rapidly when organic deficiencies are present = indicator drop (ID.).

5.7.

When diagnosing the function of the main internal organs, four consecutive measurement points on the meridians of the terminal parts of the extremities have to be measured in order not to overlook an indicator drop (ID.) which may be present only on one point. Furthermore, the individual points may be used for differential diagnosis of special parts or portions of organs (see *Voll, Topographic Positions of the Measurement Points in Electro-Acupuncture,* Textual Volume I, Illustrated Volume I (1976), Illustrated Volume II (1977), Textual- and Illustrated Volume III (1976), 1st Supplement (1978) published by ML-Publisher, Uelzen).

5.

5.8.

In practice, it turned out to be useful that the patient, for measurements of acupuncture points on the feet, hold the hand-electrode in the hand on the same side of the body, on which the foot is measured (hand-electrode = tube-electrode = "inactive" electrode = negative electrode).

According to Dr. *Kuhn,* diagonal measurements (such as right hand – left foot) in elder individuals may yield slightly different measurement results in comparison to measurements taken on the same half of the body (such as right hand – right foot).

5.9.

In point measurements using optimal pressure for obtaining the maximum value, the rapidity of exercising the contact pressure has to be considered. When a pressure is increased only slowly, the actually existing maximum value cannot be reached, in that it will stay below that very value.

5.

5.10.
Graphs

5.10.1.
Relations between contact pressure and measurement results in the diagnostic part of the electro-acupuncture apparatus acc. to Voll.

1 = Pointed electrode 2 mm ∅
2 = Four pin electrode and 3 mm ball-electrode
3 = Semicircular electrode 4 mm ∅

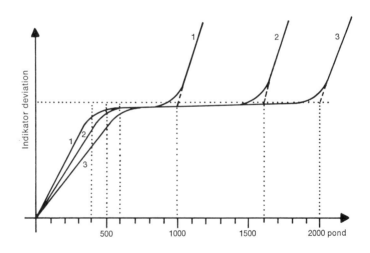

5.

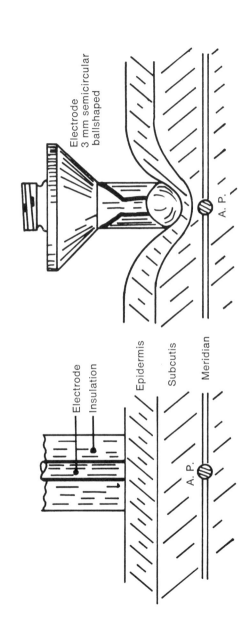

5.10.2

Measurements taken on the surface of the skin
(acc. to Croon)

Electrode
Insulation
Epidermis
Subcutis
A. P.
Meridian

5.10.3

Electro-acupuncture measurements taken with optimal pressure
(non-pathologic)

Electrode
3 mm semicircular
ballshaped
A. P.

6. How are the measurement readings evaluated?

6.1.

In order to establish a survey of all the registrated measurement values, it is recommended to write down each individual value.

Measurement result:

6.2.

The measurement value travels to the middle of the scale (50) to remain there: The reaction of the acupuncture point corresponds to normal functions. Dr. *Voll* points out that the value of 50 is an ideal value, hardly found in men today with the exception of healthy infants of several days of age or in people living remote from civilization.

6.3.

The indicator of the measurement device travels up to values above the middle of the scale and then becomes stable (50 to 100): The acupuncture point and thus the organ associated with the acupuncture point is irritated (either physiologically or already pathologically). (For evaluation of the measurement results, see 6.6.)

6.4.

The measurement value does not reach the value of 50 although one is certain to have located the acupuncture point precisely: the bio-electric energy, for some reason or other, is impeded as to its free flow, or the production of bio-electric energy is reduced such as in degenerative processes.

6.5.

The indicator exceeds a value of 50, however does not remain stable but starts dropping more or less rapidly to reach, after a time of 10 - 15 - 20 seconds, a certain lower stable point: indicator drop (ID.).

6.

6.5.1.

As mentioned above, the acupuncture point is stimulated by the electric measurement current. This outside irritation is followed by a reaction inside. A healthy body will counter the outside irritation by an equally large reaction from the inside. Thus, an equilibrium is reached in terms of the stable measurement value.

6.5.2.

When the organ to be measured is weakened to an extent that a sufficient counter-reaction to the intruding current is no longer possible, the state of equilibrium is disturbed resulting in the indicator to change its value (indicator drop). The ID. is a clear indication for an organ disturbance, in which specific cellular tissue has become insufficient. The magnitude of the indicator drop, that is, the measurement value between the maximum instable (labile) value and the final stable value is simultaneously a measure for the extent of the functional insufficiency.

6.5.3.

A slow indicator rise up to the maximum value indicates that the organ related to the acupuncture point is fatigued mobilizing its final reserves to balance the intruding current.

This organic fatigue is followed very soon by functional disturbances of the organ.

6.6.

Summary and evaluation

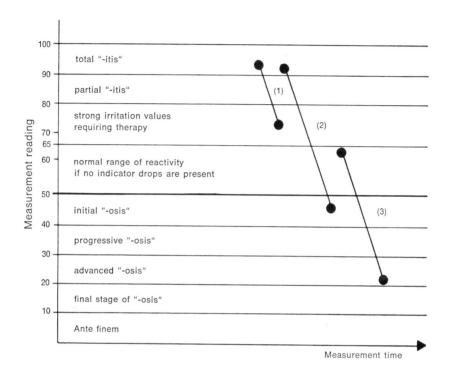

(1) = "-itis" tractable by therapy
(2) = "-osis" and superimposed "-itis" still tractable
(3) = "-osis" in peril, when indicator drop subsides below thirty.

7.

7. How is the measurement of the acupuncture point visualized?

7.1.

As outlined above, the measurement taken on an acupuncture point may be considered as an interference with the bio-electric pathways (meridians) by subtracting energy. On the acupuncture points, sensitive measurement devices possessing high internal ohmic resistances may establish a voltage exceeding by far that of the surrounding polarization voltage.

Regarding energy subtraction on the acupuncture point in man, see test carried out by *Voll* described in the Textual Volume I on page 160.

7.1.1.

By polarisation voltage is understood the voltage arising when a metal touches an ionized liquid. The bio-electric energy may be measured by approaching the pointed electrode as close to the acupuncture point as possible and by placing the counter pole as the hand or tube electrode in one hand of the patient. Thus, it may be verified that the acupuncture point possesses a negative potential while the skin of the hand shows a positive potential.

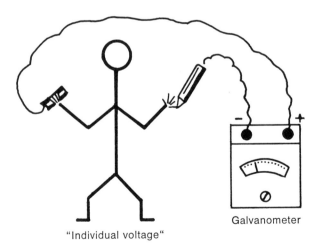

"Individual voltage"

Galvanometer

7.1.2.

7.1.2.

What is negative and positive electricity?

The electric energy is restricted (in part) to electricity carriers, also referred to as electrons. The electrons constitute negatively charged electricity particles. The negative charge of a body, therefore, results from a surplus of electrons in this specific body. In contrast, the positive charge of the body represents a lack of electrons.

7.2.

When the functional state of an acupuncture point is measured by an electric current constituting a stimulus polarized opposite to the body, the body will feel this as an "intervention" to cause its reaction.

When strong currents are used as stimuli on the body this reaction will no longer occur. The body succumbs to the stimulus and helps itself by contracting its tissues to decrease the conductivity of the skin and the muscular tissue to avoid the destructive effects of the electric currents on the body's electrolyte liquids. However, when the stimulus remains within physiologic magnitudes, that is, the body is capable of responding to the stimulus to the full extent, this will facilitate a functional diagnosis of the acupuncture point and thus, of the organ related to the acupuncture point by means of the stimulus and its counter-reaction.

7.3.

Very sensitive measurement devices using electrical currents too small for the body to respond to cannot establish diagnosis in the same sense as electro-acupuncture according to *Voll.* In such a case, no indicator drops will result, since the electric stimulus will be countered by the body or by one of its organs anyhow.

7.4.

The indicator drop is not to be considered as the result of a polarization voltage, because graphite electrodes may yield an indicator drop equally well, showing the same magnitudes (examination results by Dr. *Becker,* 1972, Euratom Ispria).

8.

8. Would it be better to use an electrode of constant pressure and would it be preferable to separate the diagnostic from the therapeutic part of the instrument?

8.1.

It should be clear from the above outlines that the application of an electrode of constant pressure would not be useful for electro-acupuncture in the daily practice. The fact alone, that in small infants the corium is sufficiently drained lymphatically, i.e., is electrically well conductible while keratosis in elder individuals increases the resistance to the electric current, clearly shows that the utilization of a foolproof, easily manipulatable and pressure-constant stylus cancels out. The acupuncture points, on a callous palm, require a larger contact pressure. Apart from this, the tolerance of the contact pressure of the electrode ranging from approx. 600 to approx. 1800 pond is so large that the utilization of an electrode of inconstant pressure is appropriate in practice for measurements taken in electro-acupuncture.

8.2.

Many speculations were made as to the usefulness of separating the two units, that is, the diagnostic and the therapeutic part to form one separate diagnostic device and one separate therapeutic device in one casing each. Experience in electro-acupuncture, however, has shown, that in order to carry out therapy with the instrument, the exact dosage of the applied low frequency current impulses require the measuring device, i.e., the diagnostic part. The therapeutic part of the instrument may equally be applied to stimulate latent odontogenic foci and to verify subsequently connections of odontogenic foci with chronic disturbances in the body. (See 11.4).

The K+F-Diatherapuncteur apparatus and all the other EAV-apparatuses have to be considered as optimal constructions, and it is only a question of the casing whether the instrument is to be accommodated in a desk-shaped, in a flat, or in any other casing.

8.

A supplementary construction in this field is the *K+F-Neuromat,* which automatically regulates the therapy of the conductance values (charging and discharging or increasing and decreasing). Thus, normotonia can always be reached. The *Neuromat* is only useful for therapy and for the constant balance of normotonia following previous and fundamental therapy. There are no objections to handing such an instrument to the patient for his personal use. The instrument can only be applied using two hand-, two foot-, or two sheet-electrodes (see also 9.1 and 9.3). Overtreatment is not possible since when decreasing (discharging), the green light turns to red and vice versa, that is, when charging or increasing, the red light changes to green.

9.

9. Which facilities are offered by the K+F-Diatherapuncteur, by the Dermatron, and by the other EAV-instruments?

Measurement facilities not associated directly with electro-acupuncture according to *Voll* are as follows:

9.1.
Measurement of the entire conductance value (hand-hand).

In this measurement, the stylus is inserted into the hand-electrode using the contact plug – in addition, there is a cable (therapy cable) fitted with two banana plugs at the ends without a stylus – thus both hand-electrodes may be connected to the cable and placed into the patient's hands. In such measurements, it turned out that the reading achieved has two range at least between 82 and 85 to make sure, that a diagnostic indicator drop cannot be overlooked. It is only when the body shows these values that its bio-electric energetic circulation is functioning guaranteeing for all indicator drops to be noticeable as indications of organic insufficiency. The value of 80 is the separation point between vagotonia and sympathicotonia. From 82 upwards the sympathicotonic state begins, and from 78 downwards, conversely, the vagotonic state is valued. Therefore, it is indispensible to carry out these hand-hand conductance value measurements prior to other electro-acupuncture measurements (see also 9.2.).

In subnormal values (vagotonic state), an adequate therapy (recharging) has to be carried out using alternating low frequency current impulses up to the tingling intensity to be discussed later on (see 23.2.).

9.2.
Measurements of quadrants.
In addition to the upper half of the body which may be measured by the hand-hand measurements, values of the lower half of the body have to be established by foot-foot-measurements (using two foot-electrodes). Apart from this, the conductance value of the right or the left half of the body may also be taken as a diagnostic hint. In this latter case, one hand- and one foot-electrode respectively are used.

9.3.

When all of these four mentioned values are equal or almost equal, we may conclude, that the body is in its autonomic energetic equilibrium, in other words in harmony. When the four quadrant measurements differ, disharmony is present. In order to increase the body's response to therapy, no matter of which kind, in other words to support the introduced therapeutic measures, it is useful as a basic therapy to balance the four quadrants of the body by charging or discharging the body using low frequency current impulses.

9.4.

In addition, there exists another possibility for applying the diagnostic part of the instrument using the so-called *Regelsberger* measurement technique on the vertebral spine. For this – like described above with respect to the measurements of the entire conductance value – the hand-electrodes are replaced by so-called roller-electrodes. One of these roller-electrodes is taken to pass along the spinous processes of the vertebral column, while the other roller-electrode is conducted parallel to that, that is, following essentially the urinary bladder meridian's course. When the skin of the back is very dry, which is frequently the case, it has to be wetted. By this measurement a pure resistance measurement is carried out, and the absolute indicator deviation of the instrument is decisive to give a maximum reading on a diseased spot. When one passes over a spot on the vertebral spine where pathologic processes are present, one obtains a larger conductivity, in other words the resistance is decreasing. We may conclude, therefore that when a rise of conductivity (of the measurement value) is obtained, pathologic conditions have to be assumed to be present at that spot. In using the roller-electrodes, we may likewise achieve indicator drops, such as in isolated diseases of vertebrae requiring further special diagnostics.

The increase of the conductance value in measurements along the vertebral spine is not achieved momentarily but tends to climb slowly to its maximum value and to decrease again. The spot showing the maximum reading has to be subjected to further analysis. Readings have to be taken separately both on the right and on the left side of the vertebral column. In addition to that, indi-

9.

vidual measurement points for the vertebral column are available, that is, the 11. Urinary bladder point, as well as for the spinal marrow, that is, the 13. Governor point (see outlines in other volumes).

Recently, the differentiated measurement points for the cervical, thoracic, and lumbar spine have been established (see *Voll:* Illustrated Volume II, Fig. 24).

9.5
Figures
Poles in quadrant derivations

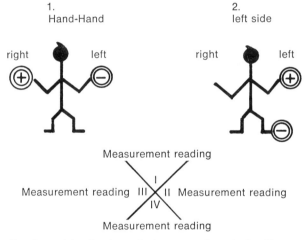

How to register the 4 conductance readings in the file

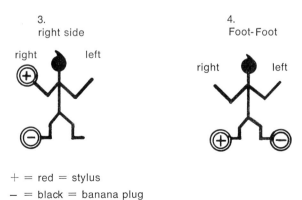

+ = red = stylus
− = black = banana plug

9.

9.6. Summarizing remarks

9.6.1.

The ideal normal value for measurements of the acupuncture point is 50 and should always be reached in therapeutic procedures.

9.6.2.

The normal value for measurements of the entire conductance value, i.e., for sheet-like measurements taken between one skin area and another skin area, has to amount to at least 82 in order for EAV-diagnostics to be complete. It is only in a state of sympathicotonia that all indicator drops (ID.) in organic insufficiencies will show.

9.6.3.

Readings taken on the Hypothalamus points after each correct and complete treatment should by all means reach values of 50. It is known, however, that this ideal value cannot be maintained for very long, since environmental influences with all their irritations and impacts tend to increase this hypothalamus value, which is also promoted by the autonomic counter-regulation. For this reason, a compromise was achieved, in that hypothalamus measurement values ranging between 50 and 65 should not be considered as pathologic values, provided the measurement readings on hands and feet remain without indicator drops below 65. When the peripheral values obtained on hands and feet lie above those taken from the hypothalamus measurement points (such as hypothalamus 74, with peripheral values more than 80) a toxic hypothalamic bloc has to be expected. One should be concerned, when the hypothalamus values show indicator drops. When these are present, a preceding commotio cerebri (concussion of the brain) or a degenerative nerve disease of the cerebrum (brain) has to be expected. The first case may also be established anamnestically. In the latter case, strong impacts of chemical or electric noxae may be present.

10.

10. What has to be considered in searching for foci (focal testing)?

10.1.

The most prominent focal disturbances occur in the area of the head, such as in teeth, in teethless jaw sections, in paranasal cavities, in tonsils, in the mastoid bone, which will simultaneously involve the central switchboard of all organic functions, the hypothalamus.

The hypothalamus measurement point is situated at the uppermost attachement of the ear, somewhat higher and backwards in an osseous pit palpable with the searching finger. When both hypothalamus values are equal on the right and left side as well as below 80, one will expect no acute odontogenic focus to be present, whereas latent foci actually may be present. When the hypothalamus exhibits values ranging between 82 to 88, foci are sure to be present.

10.2.

Since focal disturbances in chronic deseases in addition to being monofocal, will mostly occur plurifocally, the presence of the occurrence of one or several foci on the right or left side of the body has to be envisaged. When hypothalamus values range between 82 to 88 on both sides, the presence of several foci has to be concluded.

10.3.

Apart from this, the occurrence of foci is so multiple that it can only be touched briefly in this booklet. Please refer to "Foci in the Head" by *Voll,* ML-Publisher, Uelzen, 1974, German edition. In this volume, descriptions are given for diagnostics of the cranial foci with and without medication testing.

11. How to carry out focal testing?

11.1.

Prior to any focal measurement, the diagnosis of the lymph vessel points 1 to 3 has to be carried out.

11.1.

The following lymph vessel points (Ly.) furnish clues as to the presence of foci or fields of disturbance when an indicator drop is present:

1. Ly. relating to the palatine tonsil or, in tonsillectomated individuals, to the peri- and retro-tonsillar space
1a. Ly. relating to the tubal tonsil
2. Ly. relating to the jaws
3. Ly. relating to the paranasal cavities,

just to mention the most important ones. See also *Voll:* Topographic Positions of the Measurement Points in Electro-Acupuncture, Illustrated Volume II, Fig. 5.

11.2.

When one suspects a dental focus because of an indicator drop on the 2. Lymph vessel point, the six jaw measurement points have to be checked following the diagram below as to the corresponding odontons: (In addition Textual and Illustrated Volume III shows and describes measurement points for the ten jaw sections on Figures 18, 19 and 20).

	7. MP. Stomach	25. MP. Governor vessel		7. MP. Stomach
upper jaw	8 – 5	4 – 1	1 – 4	5 – 8
lower jaw	8 – 5	4 – 1	1 – 4	5 – 8
	right side	midline		left side
	8. MP. Stomach	24. MP. Conception vessel		8. MP. Stomach

11.

11.2.1.

The measurement point for the upper incisors 1 to 4 on the left and right side is situated upwards on the governor vessel (25. Governor vessel point) almost in the midposition between the base of the tip of the nose and the upper lip. This point referring to the lower jaw is situated on the so-called conception vessel (24. Conception vessel point) in the dimple below the lower lip.

11.2.2.

The measurement points pertaining to the lateral parts of the jaws for the odontons 5 to 8 are situated at 135 degrees respectively, projecting upwards for the upper jaw and approx. 1/4 FB (FB = finger breadth = 2nd phalanx of the middle finger between the ends of the articular creases when the finger is bent rectangularly) off the angle of the mouth for the lower jaw, the distance for the upper jaw being slightly larger than that for the lower one.

Note: in a small mouth the relative distance is larger as to the angle of the mouth.

11.3.

Jaw measurement points showing values ranging between 90 and 92 without showing indicator drops may exhibit the following irritations: Several metals may be present forming an electric element in contact with the saliva, that is, produce a voltage and an electric current, disturbing the bio-electric situation in the oral cavity. This may be verified by using the "Potential Measurement Device".

– Inflammatory processes in the gingiva may be present (serous inflammation, such as in allergic irritations).

11.4.

In order to locate a focus exactly, the jaw measurement point related to the focus has to be decreased by low frequency positive current impulses of least intensity down to the value of 50. This may be difficult at times but will be successful when one keeps on decreasing. This will be indicated by the hypothalamus value and the 2. Lymph measurement point to show decreasing values as well. When this is the case one will take the tooth electrode, that is, by placing the plexiglas elongation piece on top of the ball-electrode, to apply a slight current impulse on each tooth root in succession (intensity 20 in the Diatherapuncteur apparatus. Intensity 3 in the Dermatron apparatus using a frequency of 10 Hertz). After each current impulse a reading is taken on the respective tooth measurement point and on the 2. Lymph measurement point. The tooth root yielding an elevated measurement reading after electrical stimulation on the jaw measurement point and the 2. Lymph vessel point has to be considered as being focated. This procedure may be repeated by decreasing the jaw measurement points intermittently down to 50 until all of the roots have been tested to show that on one side – even in the toothless jaw – there may be several foci present. (See "Foci in the Head" ML-Publisher 1974, German edition, pages 91, 92 and 219.)

11.5.

The other acupuncture points known on the head have to be evaluated as well.

11.6.1.

Special nosodes for verifying kind and extent of a focus:

Nosode of chronic pulpitis
nosode of gangrenous pulp
nosode of granuloma of the tooth root
nosode of radicular cyst
nosode of follicular cyst
nosode of jaw ostitis
nosode of necrotizing ostitis
nosode of exudative ostitis
nosode of tooth pocket

11.6.2.

Diagnosis of the extent (serverity) of a focus using various potencies

D 10			incipient focal
D 8			disturbances
D 6	1:	1 000 000	initial focal disturbances
D 5	1:	100 000	developing focal
D 4	1:	10 000	disturbances

11.

D	3	1 ampule	1× 1 :	1 000	strong focus
D	3	2 ampules	2× 1 :	1 000	stronger focus
D	3	3 ampules	3× 1 :	1 000	very strong focus
D	3	4 ampules and more	1 :	1 000	extremely strong focus (for surgical treatment)

12.

12. How does electro-acupuncture diagnosis differ from other known electrical diagnostic procedures?

12.1

Electro-acupuncture diagnosis is based on sending direct current obtained from a current source of high internal resistance through the body using an exactly calibrated magnitude derived from a phantom for every instrument.

12.2.

Measurements carried out by this direct current as a stimulus is a functional test just strong enough to provoke a healthy body to bring about a state of equlibrium between the stimulus and its own reaction (stable value).

12.3.

When the supplied magnitude of current administered to the body is too small, a sufficient counter reaction on the part of the body will always be achieved to cope with the intruding current. A super-sensitive instrument, therefore, will not yield an indicator drop even if an organic disturbance is present. When larger quantities of current are passed through the body, larger than the body can cope with, there will always be an indicator drop present (coarse measurement instrument). In this case the body will not be able to bring about any counter-reaction. It is the achievement of electro-acupuncture to have found out about the proper calibration of the electric stimulation to achieve a marginal magnitude between the reaction of the healthy and the pathologic situation.

12.4.

Other methods known to the author, essentially apply alternating current *(Croon)* of high frequency in order to avoid the very phenomenon of the indicator drop, which cannot always be achieved. Furthermore, *Croon's* method derives the measurement values from the surface of the skin rather than from the deeper layers of the skin like electro-acupuncture does.

12.

12.5.

The indicator drop was established for the first time by Dr. *W. Schmidt,* München, by means of an instrument using alternating current of 50 Hertz. He described this phenomenon in 1952. This instrument, however, took a long time to achieve the complete indicator drop, i.e., to reach the minimal stable value. This is why in practical applications this instrument is considered to be too time consuming. Therefore it did not gain any larger range of applications.

12.6.

Dr. *de la Fuye,* as mentioned above, combined the inserted acupuncture needle with an electrical therapeutic instrument (see page 28). According to his own statements, however, he could not achieve any practical measurement results for diagnostics.

12.7.

In recent years, a large number of acupuncture instruments of various design have been thrown on the market. It has to be pointed out that only those apparatuses and instruments described in this booklet have been examined by Dr. *Voll* and his colleagues and were approved to carry out electro-acupuncture according to *Voll.* Only these apparatuses may be called "EAV-instruments".

13.

13. How about the scientific evidence of acupuncture points and meridians?

13.1.

The pathologist is not able to prove the existence of acupuncture and its meridians, because it is the bio-electric energy in the living tissue only which can be measured by modern biophysical means (see page 42).

13.2.

Special achievements have also been reached by Dr. *Niboyet* who proved that the human skin contains points varying in their electrical properties as to their surroundings. He also tried to send direct current through the skin taken from the body and derive it at other places of the skin characterized by the above mentioned meridians and acupuncture points.

14.

14. How does electro-acupuncture therapy differ from electrical therapy using different kinds of instruments?

14.1.

Those therapy instruments known to the author employ essentially pure sinusoidal alternating currents of high frequency or frequencies between 50 and 100 Hertz, also combinations of the two.

14.2.

Therapy carried out by the *K + F-Diatherapuncteur* or the other EAV-instruments may be divided into two principles:

14.2.1.

Principles acting on the acupuncture points: Acupuncture points may be charged by alternating currents of higher intensity, thus rendering them more conductible. When direct current of low intensity is used the resistance of the acupuncture point may be raised, that is "decreased". In electro-acupuncture diagnosis (diagnostic therapy) the value is decreased to 50 (discharging) or raised up to 50 (charging).

14.2.2.

Differing from this, measurements of the entire conductance value are carried out. In individual point stimulations we treat the corresponding organ or, when several points are stimulated on the same meridian, several parts of the organ in order to achieve normotonia or normergia. However, in the holistic treatment by means of the hand- or foot-electrodes via the four quadrants

I.	right and left hand	HH
II.	left hand left foot	LS
III.	right hand and right foot	RS
IV.	right and left foot	FF

we may re-establish a disturbed harmony by employing the so-called alternating (charging) or direct current (discharging) relaxation oscillations (see also page 93). For this, it is assumed that each organ in the human body possesses a low frequency of its own. When we know the frequency which belongs to the state of harmony, we may choose this specific frequency in the therapy part of the EAV-instrument, add the missing frequency to cause a resonance absorption of the diseased organ, and stimulate the own production of this frequency.

The "wave swing" or "wave sweep", as an automatic change of frequencies back and forth between 0.8 to 10.0 Hertz, facilitates the application of this resonance frequency to the body, which in turn may pick its proper frequency in order to re-establish its live functions. In other words: The relaxation oscillations applied by the K + F-Diatherapuncteur or by the EAV-instruments have a spasmolytic and tonifying effect. The application of relaxation oscillations also enables the body to have a normal tonic flux of its bioelectric energy. Further outlines on this may be found in the paper: Twenty years of Electro-acupuncture Therapy using low-frequency current pulses (Am. J. Acupuncture, Vol. 3, Nr. 4, Oct.–Dec. 1975, pages 205–296).

14.2.3.

Patients exhibiting total conductance values on all four quadrants far below a normal value of 82 may be applied the neccessary energy in the following fashion (according to Kuhn):

– The patient is applied the electric energy from the instrument simultaneously via the hand electrodes (hand-hand) and the foot electrodes (foot-foot) by simultaneously depressing the keys HH and FF (that is I and IV in the Dermatron).

– The patient is connected to the K + F-Diatherapuncteur instrument of older design by means of the twin cord (lead) in the usual manner to be charged (red banana plug right, black banana plug left) on hands as well as feet.

– The sufficient application (normalization) has to be checked separately both for HH and FF.

14.2.4.

A combination of these two therapeutic methods (that is 14.2.1. and 14.2.2.) is made possible by using the "wave swing" according to item 14.2.1. (Electro-acupuncture diagnosis and therapy).

14.

14.3.

Recent investigations have shown, that a "negative direct current relaxation oscillation", i.e. negative sawtooth, will rapidly create a higher conductance of the acupuncture point. This has to be visualized as a local charging of the acupuncture point (accumulator effect). The re-establishment of the bio-electric energy flow postulated by *Voll*, that is, changing the static state to the dynamic state, can only be reached by applying a major amount of energy (strong stimulus) over a longer period of time. In patients suffering from pronounced energy deficiency, the "negative sawtooth" should be used as a pre-treatment, using the alternating relaxation oscillation with just bearable tingling intensity as an after-treatment. (See furthermore page 96.)

15. How can relaxation oscillations be applied to the body?

15.1.

The simplest way of applying these relaxation oscillations to the body is by means of hand and foot electrodes. This procedure is useful for the treatment of the four quadrants correspondingly in order to reach a value of at least 82 on the respective half of the body (increasing or decreasing), in addition to establishing the conductance values on the respective quadrant. For decreasing (discharging), it should be noted that in starting from high initial values, one sometimes can achieve only a decrease of the indicator reading by two to four units on the scale.

When, after an initial lowering, the conductance value starts climbing again, the treatment has to be finished immediately. That is why one should always control the conductance value when one applies decreasing (discharging) therapy, in order to recognize a reversed rising of the indicator (possibly use key for automatic control in *Dermatron*).

15.2.

In chronic articular diseases, in which one joint exhibits widely differing conductance values, the utilization of two roller-electrodes or, alternatively, of two sheet electrodes turned out to be useful. The fact that both electrodes are applied to a milieu of poor electric conductivity enables one to locally use higher energy, without these electric currents causing discomfort to the patient.

15.3.

Apart from this, electrodes for gynaecology (vaginal electrodes of various sizes) are available as well as a rectal electrode for anal treatment in women and men (or for treatments of the prostate in men) supplied with a notch and an insulation part for the sphincter of the anus with the metal part being gilded because of the presence of aggressive mucous secretions of the large intestine.

For treating hip complaints in women, it is recommended to use the vaginal electrode, while in men one should insert the rectal electrode, placing the second electrode as a sheet electrode on the hip joint itself.

15.

15.4.

The intensity to be applied should be such that it does not hurt the patient beyond the tingling intensity, which is considered ideal. The patient should be in a position to rid himself of the electrical treatment or decrease the intensity, in particular, when it turns out that an initial low conductance value with a slight effect only of the electric current on the sensitive nervous system may be followed by an increased susceptibility to the current in the course of the treatment. As the conductance value increases, the flow of the current may reach such magnitudes as to cause considerable discomfort to the patient. When this is present, it is a proof for the efficacy of the relexation oscillations and should be noted in any case.

15.5.

The therapeutic part of the apparatus, moreover, is used to irritate latent foci by applying the electrical current (see chapter 11.4.) to them.

15.5.1.

Used in the entire jaw area for the activation of latent foci.

For this, one uses a stylus made out of plexiglass together with a tooth-electrode, instead of using the hand-electrode (stylus).

The normal stylus is mounted with an elongation piece including the tooth-electrode. On both sides, between teeth 8+ to +8 and 8− to −8* a current impulse is applied buccal-palatinally and buccal-lingually using an intensity of approx. 20 scale units (per cent indicator deviation) in the $K + F$-Diatherapuncteur or three scale units in the Dermatron apparatus for a duration of approx. 0,5 seconds. Turn on: Increasing (charging), and 10 Hertz by "hand". Furthermore, as described above with respect to the location of foci.

15.5.2.

For individual teeth:

For this, an elongation piece including a tooth-electrode is

---

* in the American nomenclature 1 to 16 and 17 to 32

mounted on the stylus. The other electrode, that is, the hand-electrode as counter electrode, is placed in the patient's hand in the usual way.

Turn on: Increasing (charging) using 10 Hertz with key "hand" depressed, intensity as described above.

Then a short current impulse is applied to the root to be examined, i.e., buccally, lingually, or palatinally. When a subsequent reading on the tooth measurement point and on the 2. Lymph measurement point yields measurement values of more than 80 plus indicator drop, this is sufficient evidence for the latent focus to be activated, which is thus confirmed.

15.6.

In the ophthalmic area one should keep off the eyes at a distance of one hand breadth (generally speaking) using only direct current relaxation oscillations (decreasing) since otherwise the eye nerves may be irritated too strongly and light flashes may be seen by the patient. The intensity should be adapted to the patient's discretion when he still feels it to be pleasant. This, for example, is important for rolling the cheeks using the narrow roller-electrode, for trigeminal neuralgia (Dr. *Oltrogge*).

15.7.

When the body resists the electrical treatment to a major extent, in particular in treatments of the periostium and of tendons, it may turn out to be useful for quick help to carry out a so-called moxa treatment. For this, the instrument is turned on maximum intensity using a frequency of 10 Hertz and placing the hand-or roller-electrode on the area to be treated. The counter electrode should be placed as close to the area to be treated as possible. The knob on the stylus is then depressed for one second, thus applying a short current on the energetically deficient area and causing the spastic bloc to be interrupted at this place (maximum treatment).

16.

16. Which frequencies are chosen for therapy?

16.1.

One form of application of relaxation oscillations for the human body is the so-called wave swing, also referred to as wave sweep. By means of an electronic device incorporated in the *K + F-Diatherapuncteur* the frequencies, i.e., the oscillations per second, are changed two times each three minutes from 0.8 to 10.0 Hertz back and forth. The *Dermatron* apparatus starts at 0.8 to reach 10 Hertz re-iterating this procedure. In the *Dermatron*, the following keys are used for operation: WS not depressed. Small toggle switch turned from "D" to "T". Subsequently, choise of current characteristic and intensity.

16.2.

For specific therapy, it is useful to apply specific frequencies. These frequencies may be turned on and read by means of a so-called ten-spiral-pontentiometer. In the "Dermatron" instrument a separate measurement scale is installed. The whole range for the electric formation of the frequency is not, like usually, on a potentiometer with a maximum scale deviation of 270 degrees, but rather on a potentiometer of 10 revolutions, that is 3600 degrees. Thus, it is possible to exactly turn on a specific frequency up to one to two decimals behind the comma. In the *Dermatron* apparatus the desired frequency is turned on by adjusting the dial denoted "freq" after depressing the key "hand" for the measurement scale on the right side. Empirically established frequencies may be applied as to special diseases and demands.

17. What is medication testing?

17.1.

Medication testing in electro-acupuncture has been much disputed. It is the result of a coincidence.

17.2.

Medication testing is carried out in the following manner:

17.2.1.

First of all, readings are taken from acupuncture points and, at the same time, possible indicator drops are noted, like described above. These indicator drops, as a rule, necessitate the application of medications. Then, combinations of various medications (homeopathic, biologic or herbal) or nosodes have to be determined in order to balance the acupuncture points to 50, that is, all measurement values including the hypothalamus. This procedure is referred to, after *Voll*, as mesenchyme reactivation using mainly nosodes and accompanying (complementary) homeopathic medications for drainage (see also Fundamentals of Mesenchyme reactivation in "Foci in the Head" by Dr. *Voll*, pages 237 to 266, ML-Publisher, German edition.

Toxins deposited in the mesenchyme are being transmitted to the lymphatic circulation by means of nosodes. Furthermore, the secreting organs have to be stimulated as to their functions in order to achieve a draining therapy. For this, please consult the compilations of nosodes and their accompanying medications to be used in medical and dental offices mentioned in various publications (see also item 17.3.).

17.2.2.

The suitable medications in ampules selected for the type of patient and his complaints are put in the patient's hand or in a medication honeycomb for testing (the honeycomb is connected to the measuring circle). The effects of the medications on a patient's system are then verified by means of the diagnostic part of the instrument. When the indicator drop has disappeared and/or measurement values got closer to normal, the correct medication has been found, which is verified by a value of 50 on the measurement scale.

As a result of medication testing, a combination of medications is established by means of all their components and dosages to achieve a balancing of the patient's previous otherwise pathologic values. See also bind 14 of the Schriftenreihe des Zentralverbandes der Ärzte für Naturheilverfahren "Medikamententestung, Nosodentherapie und Mesenchymentschlackungstherapie bzw. Mesenchymreaktivierung".

17.3.

Once again nosodes have mobilized the mesenchyme and fatty tissue to release their toxins into the blood and lymph circulation, one should make sure that these toxins are not deposited at different parts of the body.

In order to promote the secretion of all organs, it is necessary to apply accompanying (complementary) medications in the form of draining medications and have the patient take a lot of liquids during the mesenchyme reactivation cure (MRC).

18. Pre-requisites for carrying out medication testing.

18.1.

Medication testing is the most excellent achievement of electro-acupuncture. In medication testing it is obvious that very small energies, which the medication in the glass ampule conveys on to the patient, have an impact on the autonomic nervous system (somatic tissue primarily) of the patient via the acupunctural system.

18.2.

An energetic influence between person to person is likewise known (according to *Schick*, oral communication, and others). When one, as a treating doctor, is subjected to any pathologic disturbances, these disturbances will be conveyed to the patient thus rendering medication testing to yield faulty values. It is, therefore, recommended to have the doctor's body under control by applying electro-acupuncture every day thus coping with possible disturbances immediately. This may not always be easy and sometimes even requires the cooperation of medical colleagues for complete therapy, or in dental problems, of the dentist for dental defocation. Current checks may be carried out by the doctor on himself, of course. In severe pathologic alterations one should use only cotton gloves *(Kuhn)* or, preferably, a linen handkerchief wrapped around the hands thus avoiding any direct contact with a patient in medication testing.

18.3.

In any case, it is considered useful to protect the one hand in contact with the patient as described above, that is, not in charge of holding the stylus *(Kuhn)*, in order to avoid an energy transfer from the examiner to the patient and vice versa. This is, in particular, required for examiners suffering from wet skin. Furthermore, it is essential, that the patient, while being tested, is not subjected to any influences from outside such as electric fields etc. (see also item 21.7.).

18.

18.4.

In many cases, outsiders emphasize the so-called geopathic irritational zones. I do not doubt, that there do exist influences on the body caused by natural influences, by the earth and by the sky. The earth possesses an electrical field, which changes constantly. Likewise, the earth possesses a magnetic field, which may be influenced with respect to its intensity by outside forces. The body of the earth itself is composed inhomogenously, which has an impact both on the electrical and on the magnetic field. However, we are born into this world of "geopathy" and need these charges for training our autonomic nervous system and for balancing our bioelectric energy *(Kneipp)*. We know, that a person living permanently in a faradic cage, will become sick. There have even been fatal incidences, when e.g. actresses had applied a metallic coating on their skin: The short circuit of their bio-electric energy and the lack of recharging from outside caused death: In addition, the impeded breathing of the skin naturally played an important roll as well.

Still worse seem to me the disturbances caused by modern buildings (faradic cages) because of their intensive electric installations (electric alternating fields of 50 Hertz). These alternating fields have such a disturbing impact on the human body, in particular on sleep, that neural distonia may easily be caused. According to my personal opinion, it is much more important for patients to live in a climate healthy for sleep and to be able to work at a place free from low frequency alternating fields.

See also: *Werner:* Suggestions for biologically adoquato Building, 1976, ML-Publisher, Uelzen, Germany.

18.6.

Kuhn emphasizes that patients being tested for diagnosis should constantly "try to relax" in order to avoid faulty measurements due to contractions.

19.

19. Is there any scientific proof for medication testing?

19.1.

The exact physical proof about the effective mechanism of medication testing cannot be given so far according to our physical methods known. In many tests Dr. *Morell* has verified the influence on the blood sedimentation rate caused by tested mediacations after prior injection. When medication testing had been carried out properly, blood sedimentation was improved by 20 to 40 per cent. This method could be confirmed by various electro-acupuncture doctors.

19.2.

Personally, I can confirm this on the bases of measurements taken on patients with the aid of an R-C-measurement device, prior to and after testing, resulting in obvious differences in the measurement values. The same results could be obtained by Prof. *Kracmar,* the inaugurator of the R-C-measurement method together with Dr. *Kollmer* and Dr. *Voll.* See also: "Medication testing, Nosodetherapy and Mesenchyme reactivation", ML-Publisher, 1976, German edition.

19.3.

Dr. *Höllischer* reports on: "Physical Observations related to the Problem of Medication Testing according to Voll", in which he used the electro-neural procedure according to *Croon* by means of somagrams and the infra-red procedure according to *Schwamm* to prove these relations. Furthermore, Dr. *Glaser-Türk* in *Voll's* book "Foci in the Head" reports on "The Annulation of the Electro-Cutaneous-Test (ECT) by means of Electro-Acupuncture Medication Testing" which may serve as a further proof for justifying medication testing.

19.4.

Many of Dr. *Voll's* co-workers report in his book: "Medication Testing, Nosodetherapy and Mesenchyme Reactivation" about results in treating patients by means of tested nosodes, which is a further

19.

documentary proof for the empirical correctness of medication testing and its effects.

19.5.

In many of his other publications Dr. *Voll* reports about experiments to exclude and annihilate medication testing and its results, in order to give negative proofs of exclusion. See: "Gelöste und ungelöste Probleme der Elektroakupunktur-Diagnostik und -Therapie", ML-Publisher, Uelzen, German edition, and "Anderthalb Jahrzehnte", page 241 ff.

19.6.

Beisch reports about tests carried out to objectify pulse diagnosis by means of oscillographic registrations. Also this procedure made evident the effects of tested medications. Even balancing by means of relaxation oscillation treatments (balancing of all acupuncture points to 50) could be registered as leading to normergia. (See: "Quantification of Traditional Chinese Energy by Pulse Oscillography. One means for proving medication testing in electro-acupuncture according to *Voll*." This book will appear at the end of this year in the ML-Publishing Company).

20. Which accessories to the electro-acupuncture instruments according to Voll are obtainable?

20.1.

Each instrument is supplied with: Two hand electrodes and one stylus together with its cord (lead). The basic accessories of electrodes to be fitted to the stylus are: Two tooth-electrodes, one elongation piece for protruding into cavities of the body such as nose and throat, which may be desinfected without being heated, one ball-electrode of 3 mm diameter, one contact pflug, one four-pin-electrode, and one insulated semi-circular-electrode of 4 mm diamater for the measurement of the hypothalamus to avoid contact with the auricle.

20.2.

Not included in the normal accessories but available at any time:

20.2.1.

Wheel electrodes

20.2.2.

Roller-electrodes 4 and 8 cm broad, unipolar, paired to carry out the so-called *Regelsberger's* procedure on the vertebral spine (see item 9.4.) in addition to bipolar roller-electrodes for painful dermal areas. The bipolar roller-electrode requires only one hand for operation.

20.2.3.

Sheet electrodes for super-imposition and long lasting treatment, such as in subluxations, distortions and hematomas, as well as thrombosis and thrombophlebitis. In the latter cases equal polarity has to be strictly observed in placing the electrodes, that is, the red plug of the connecting cord (positive pole) connected with the sheet-electrode should always be placed on the painful location, in particular when repeating the treatment. Otherwise, there is danger for parts of thrombi breaking loose (risk of embolia).

20.

Electrodes have to be wetted and, for hygienic reasons, should be surrounded by a wet piece of cotton, wool, or cotton tissue as an underlayer together with rubber straps or elastic bands to be fixed to the body.

One should make sure however, not to use two wetted electrodes to be attached by one elastic band only, since in this case the current would circuit through the elastic band and not through the body. For dermal areas without hairs, therapy may be carried out using a sheet-electrode made of conductible plastic material.

Advantage: It may fit the body exactly.

Disadvantage according to *Voll*: A conductance value cannot be taken with it.

20.2.4.

Vaginal electrodes in three sizes for the application of relaxation oscillations in the vagina in gynaecologic treatments with the counter-electrode being placed on the small of the back or on the abdomen.

20.2.5.

Rectal electrodes. These electrodes have been gilded to avoid an attack on the material by the intestinal mucous. They are fitted with an insulated groove to be encircled by the sphincter of the anus in order to avoid the extrusion of the electrode during treatment. To be used for example in complaints of the prostate, rectum, and anus.

20.2.6.

One of the most important electrodes, in particular for selftreatment, are foot electrodes: Two brass sheets insulated on one side to be placed on the floor and fitted with a socket for the connection of banana plugs.

20.2.7.

For treatment, one does not have to use all these electrodes connected to the stylus and its weight, which would be in the way. Instead, one may use a shielded cable fitted on the one side with a six prong plug for the insertion into the instrument, and on the other side with two banana plugs with the black plug representing the negative and the red plug the positive pole (therapy cord).

In addition, a double therapy cord (shielded) is available being fitted with the six prong plug on the one side and two red and two black banana plugs respectively on the other side (see also 14.2.3.). Such a cord (lead) is only used for an older model of an instrument lacking the four quadrant derivations.

Note:

The *Dermatron* apparatus is supplied with cord (lead) as a normal accessory similar to the above mentioned therapy cord (not when using the *"Variopit"*). This cord serves for point finding and may not be used for applying therapy. Therefore, a red point is attached to the six prong plug. For the therapy of large areas, one of the cords may be used, reserved otherwise for the so-called four-quadrant diagnosis and -therapy (20.3.).

20.2.8.

In complying with requests of dentists a so-called gingiva electrode out of stainless steel has been made. It can be screwed on to the stylus. It has a long thin shaft of approx. 6 cm length being fitted in the front with a bulge for the treatment of the surroundings of inflamed gingiva areas, extremity wounds, and the like in electro-acupuncture.

20.2.9.

The four-pin-electrode is particularly useful for the measurement of the jaw measurement points and the measurement points of the paranasal sinuses. After wetting this electrode, it may penetrate through the insulating layers of cosmetics attached to the skin of the face, to reach a final measurement value after 3 to 4 measurements. The four-pin-electrode is also useful in men, who use after-shave lotion to tan their skins.

20.2.10.

Finally, the 0.2 or 0.3 mm ear electrode should be mentioned for the use in auricular acupuncture both for diagnosis and therapy when applying low frequency current impulses of the EAV-instruments.

20.

20.3.

In order to have a simple way of carrying out conductance measurements in addition to applying relaxation oscillation therapy, measurements and therapeutic means for the four quadrants were provided for the EAV instruments:

I. hand-hand	(HH)
II. left hand – left foot	(LS)
III. right hand – right foot	(RS)
IV. foot-foot	(FF)

using hand and foot electrodes.

By depressing the corresponding keys the various combinations may be applied, such as HH and FF simultanously (see also 14.2.3. second paragraph).

How to operate the EAV-instruments is intensively discussed in seminars and when an instrument is acquired, may also be learnt in the instructions for use (Coperational manual).

21.

21. Which kinds of disturbances may arise to impede a proper utilization of the electro-acupuncture apparatuses according to Voll?

In seminars and workshops one is usually told what the $K + F$-*Diatherapuncteur* and the other EAV-instruments effectively can do. Now I should like to mention some items in pointing out the limitations for the work in electro-acupuncture.

21.1.

Electro-acupuncture is based on classical Chinese acupuncture. Therefore, it is necessary to deal intensively with the locations of the points, with the significance of the points, and the interrelations between the various points. In electro-acupuncture, correct point finding is indispensable. It had sometimes been mentioned that the proper locations of the points in using a stylus of the $K + F$-*Dia-therapuncteur* is not so important in comparison to inserting needles. This, however, is totally wrong. In contrast to needle therapy in which the silver needle may be inserted into the halo of the acupuncture point in a situation of excess energy, the acupuncture point in electro-acupuncture diagnostics has to be located in its center in order to achieve the important criterion of an indicator drop. When using gold needles in acupuncture, the needle has to be inserted into the center of the acupuncture point since otherwise a sufficiently tonifying effect may not be reached in a situation of energetic deficiency, when there is almost no halo energetically around the acupuncture point.

In order to measure the acupuncture point exactly the point has to be contacted precisely by the tip of the test stylus. Conversely, when the point is not contacted properly, the measurement value will be misleading. This is evidenced by the fact that in the so-called "decreasing" (discharging) of the points, the reverse effect may be reached in that an "increase" (charging) of the measurement values is achieved. This is so because the electrical current, via the intercellular liquids of the subcutaneous tissue between the place of contact and the acupuncture point, finds itself a pathway of its

21.

own. For this, a certain period of time is required and only after the expiration of 10 to 20 seconds one will be able to establish a sufficiently proper measurement of the acupuncture point. It is better, of course, to contact the point correctly in the first place!

21.2.

An essential requirement for the proper execution of electro-acupuncture diagnosis is the adequate application of the contact pressure, apart from the proper point location, as mentioned above. Like the surgeon, with respect to his knife, and the dentist, with respect to his drill, the electro-acupuncturist has to learn to apply the stylus on the acupuncture point using optimal pressure. In normally lymphated skin the contact pressure from 0 to approx. 500 pond of a 3 mm ball-electrode will make the measurement value rise slowly to remain largely constant. Only when the pressure is increased to phathologic magnitudes, that is, when the stylus pierces the outer skin which happens at about 2.0 kilopond, the value will rise again rapidly. So, there is a relatively large scope for variation of the contact pressure in that you can read the value of the acupuncture point on the meter scale of the *K + F-Dia-therapuncteur* or the other EAV-apparatuses (see also paragraph 5.8.).

It is evident, that in measuring well-lymphated infantile skin the pressure need not be as high as in "tanned" skin; this is only why the stylus of constant pressure has turned out to be useless.

For better point location each instrument is supplied with a buzzer, which will reach a high pitch when the stylus has hit the point exactly. The beginner should use the 3 mm ball electrode for measurements, while the more advanced electro-acupuncturist should use the pointed electrode of 2 mm semi-circular diameter for quick use and little contact pressure. The pointed electrodes, however, are liable to risks in that they may hurt the skin.

The "Dermatron" apparatus, EAV-diagnosis in addition to using a buzzer (with highest pitch on the acupuncture point), contains another facility for point finding. For this, the so-called "point finding cord" attached to a plexiglass stylus is supplied together with every instrument. (The six prong plug is marked with a red point). The maximum indicator deviation on the measurement instrument will then show the location of the acupuncture point when stroking the skin with the electrode without using pressure. (See also operation manual of the Pitterling-Electronic Co.).

Another novelty in this respect is the *"Variopit"*. According to the instructions of Pitterling-Electronic, the acupuncture point may be located by a chain of lights in the measurement stylus when stroking across the skin lightly; following this, the measurement value may be read on the measurement instrument after applying the contact pressure as usual.

21.3.

When the bio-electric or energetic condition in the patient has turned pathologic, i.e., has worsened, it is evident that a pathologic electro-acupuncture reading will result. Prior to the establishment of every diagnosis, the total conductance value has to be verified. This is done by placing the hand-electrodes which are attached to the diagnostic part of the instrument, into each hand of the patient. The measurement value reached has to show a value of at least 82 on the scale. When the measurement value is lower, it has to be increased up to a value of at least 82 by "recharging" therapy.

When one of the four quadrants exhibits a conductance value of below 80, this value must be recharged to values of up to 82 to 84, before point measurements can be done.

21.4.

A further mistake making proper diagnosis impossible is the omission of measuring all four incipient or terminal extremity points of the meridians. According to *Voll* each point on the meridian is related to certain portions or areas of an organ. An organ need not be totally insufficient with respect to its functions.

An organic damage evident by means of an indicator drop, may not be detected unless at least the above mentioned four terminal or initial points have been measured.

It is the very achievement of electro-acupuncture to be able to establish a holistic, that is, an overall and complete diagnosis. Although this requires only relatively short time, it would be inadequate because of "lack of time", to examine only few organs. For

21.

medication testing following the establishment of a diagnosis it is important to consider all points in order to achieve an optimal therapeutic effect. This is also shown by the fact that the rate of blood sedimentation turns back to normal on injecting the tested medications, based on a comprehensive medication test *(Morell)*.

Note: The measurement of the control measurement points gives diagnostic hints as to whether or not a pathologic disturbance is present, for example in the stomach. When this can be ruled out, the four terminal or initial measurement points of the organ need not be measured. In comparing the measurement values of the control measurement points, the largest functional disturbance present in an organ may immediately be established. As to the stomach, this is shown in Illustrated Volume II, Figures 34 to 36.

21.5.

When carrying out diagnosis and therapy on other persons, you should also be able to stabilize your own labile autonomic values by self-treatment. When you suffer from foci, have your foci removed. When you suffer from chronical ailments treat them using additionally tested medications. One should always be aware, that due to the direct contact between patient and physician, one may contract some of the pathologic energy of the patient to influence one's own body. You may occasionally observe that the testing of a seriously ill patient will tire you enormously as an indication of this form of influence. It is recommended, therefore, that you treat yourself daily using the electro-acupuncture apparatus to balance your points, in addition to being administered the proper medications; also try several times a day by means of the wave swing and the four quadrant therapy to re-equilibrate your autonomic system. Insulate yourself from the patient by using cotton gloves or linen handkerchiefs.

21.6.

Another possibility for being unsuccessful is the over-treatment in using the elecro-acupuncture instrument. The therapy currents should not cause discomfort on the part of the patient. This is a basic tenet to be watched carefully. The patient should be allowed at any time to free himself from the therapy currents when these

21.

cause discomfort, should you or your assistant be unable to survey the course of the therapy or to diminish the intensity.

21.7.

Finally, electrical fields of high or low frequency may impede the proper application of electro-acupuncture procedures. A healthy person is capable of counter-regulation with respect to irritations impinging from outside. Electrical fields can only affect the body, when its bio-electric potential is either extremely low (ranging about 100 millivolts) or extremily high (ranging about 2 volts only).

The first case arises in considerable exhaustion or in older sick people while asleep. A rise of the bio-electric voltage up to 2 volts occurs only in extreme excitement, when the acupuncture points will show values of more than 100 on the measurement scale.

In measuring persons, one should be aware that an additional charge caused by electrical fields of the mains, by transformers of fluorescent lamps, by the voltage production of X-rays, ozone, or even tv-sets may lead to an indicator drop down to a value of 24 on the meter scale when patients are in bad shape, that is, an indicator drop not corresponding to the actual pathologic conditions may occur. In any case, one has to keep the examination place for your patients free from the above mentioned fields. I have discussed these problems in a little booklet entitled "Suggestions for Biologically Adequate Building" (ML-Publisher, Uelzen, 1976) in German.

22.

22. Which influence has the wetting of the electrodes?

22.1.

First of all, it should be made clear that two measurement values may be compared with each other only when they were produced under equal conditions. When this requirement could not be met, the subsequent evaluation has to take this into consideration in any case.

22.2.

Measurement readings should not be taken from injured or inflamed skin.

22.3.

We have to differ between measurements in the following fashion:

22.3.1.

When measuring the acupuncture points we have emphasized, that the ohmic resistance of the corium and the underlying skin has to be overcome in order to achieve a measurement value comparable with equal measurement conditions. It turned out to be useful to coat the stylus-electrode with a thin film of moisture prior to the point measurement. This is done by holding the tip of the stylus-electrode into a wetted pad of cotton cloth or tissue. The pad is wetted by tap-water, not by aqua destillata or by physiologic saline solution NaCl).

It should, furthermore, be stressed that the inactive electrode (hand-electrode) should be surrounded by a wet tissue, 10 cm broad, which allows the examiner to use less pressure in point measurements.

22.3.2.

In the measurement of the conductance value, this is a different matter; in contrast to the electro-acupuncture point measurement, no reactive response is measured but a resistance only (bodily resistance, not skin resistance alone).

22.

It is of major importance to have the electrode surrounded by wet tissue in order for the contact resistance between hand-electrode and skin of the patient to be minimal.

Patients suffering from dry skin, that is, bad energetic supply of the palm due to weakness of the pancreas, will not be recognized as such when the electrodes are wetted or surrounded by tissue. This is why the electrode should be dry for the evaluation of the conductance value.

22.4.

It may happen occasionally that the resistance of the skin against charging is so high (pathologic), that it would require a long time for dry electrodes to influence the body. For this reason the electrodes may be more or less wet in order to enable the electric current to stimulate the body and to cause a corresponding reaction. But this is the exception.

However, the body is only responsive to electro-acupuncture diagnostics when dry (see the above translator's note) electrodes yield useful measurement readings (conductance value more than 82).

22.5.

Sweaty skin will not yield proper measurement values. In this case, the patient should calm down. Prior to the measurement sweat should be removed from the measurement points by tissue. If necessary, the general diagnosis has to account for wet or for dry skin. In some cases, washing the hands or the lower arm thoroughly with cold water may be useful.

It also turned out to be useful to decrease elevated values in over-excited patients by means of inactive electrodes (hand electrodes) using direct current positive relaxation oscillations with least intensity up to the moment when the patient starts yawning spontaneously.

23.

23. Which operations have to be carried out successively for precise electro-acupuncture diagnosis and therapy?

23.1.
Checking the instrument:

23.1.1.
Are the electric sockets sufficiently grounded? An expert should investigate this. It may occasionally happen that grounding is insufficient.

23.1.2.
After connecting the instrument with the socket of the mains, the control lamp should shine up indicating that the instrument is turned on.

23.1.3.
Is the accumulator of the *Dermatron* machine fully loaded? Do the dry batteries of the EAV-instruments still yield sufficient power?

23.1.4.
Can the value of 100 of the diagnostic part of the instrument be reached by short circuiting the two electrodes or by adjusting the dial "100"? Is the resting position of the indicator of the diagnostic part of the instrument on position "0" when the electrodes do not touch each other? For adjustment use dial marked "0".

23.2.
First of all, the conductance value of a patient is established to verify if it is at least at 82 or more. When the measurement value remains below 80, the patient has to be charged. The patient, then, keeps the hand-electrodes in his hands or on other parts of the body to be measured. The key for "permanent therapy" is turned on. For "increasing", i.e., "charging"; the intensity potentiometer is turned to where the patient feels a slight tingling. In the *Dermatron* the toggle switch is turned on "T". The first key in the upper row for

the alternating current impulse is depressed. The intensity dial is turned up to where the patient feels a tingling.

By switching back the key for permanent therapy from "T" to "D" for diagnosis, one can check from time to time if the therapy was sufficient and if the measurement value for the conductance value climbed up to 82 or more, on the meter scale. For automatic checking, the key "automatic" may be depressed.

Usually, for this kind of therapy the "wave swing" is used. The corresponding key has to be set on "WS" for this. When "permanent therapy" is turned on, a green lamp shows up in the $K + F$-*Diatherapuncteur*. In the "Dermatron" a red light shows up in the upper right corner of the measurement scale indicating frequency.

23.3.

After checking all measurement points and establishing the momentary situation of the patient which should be noted on a sheet of paper, one should charge or discharge the individual points or test medications on them when indicator drops are present.

One should begin by measuring the lymph measurement points to verify whether or not foci are present in the head. When foci are present, one should measure and apply therapy on the cranial measurement points, followed by the points on hands and feet. By coping with the situation of cranial foci, certain organic disturbances may become less pronounced thus rendering your therapeutic efforts more effective. Here again experience is required.

23.4.

It is important that a clean hand-electrode is placed into the patient's hand, since skin- and sweat particles of the previous patient may adhere to the electrode due to the good affinity of the brass electrode to the skin. Electrodes should, therefore, be cleaned properly with water and soap and then be placed in a bowl containing water. The hand-electrodes may then be stored at a dry place. When the hand-electrode has been surrounded by cotton tissue, the cleaning is easy because of no skin and sweat particles adhering to the metal.

23.

23.5.

The cleaning of the stylus electrode is not so important, because prior to every skin contact the electrode is placed on a wetted piece of cotton, wool, or cotton tissue thus cleaning the tip of the electrode.

It may happen occassionally that the thread of the winding of the point-electrode oxydizes thus creating a contact resistance, which may falsify the measurement. This is why the winding of the electrode should also be cleaned occassionally.

23.6.

During measurements the patients should not be in contact with artificial floor covering or carpets made out of plastic materials which may possess electrostatic charges, nor should the patients be in contact with the earth. We recommend the installation of the examination place, when artificial material flooring is present, in the following manner:

23.6.1.

The floor is covered by a wire mesh consisting of zinc coated brass or iron wire depending on the local requirements as far as the area to be covered is concerned. The wire should be zinc-coated to form a homogenous conducting area without risks of terminal circuits being present. Also, a thin piece of metal sheet or copper sheet or a foil may be taken. Aluminum foil, however, causes difficulties of contact.

This mesh or metal sheet has to be well grounded. For this, the grounding of the mains or the so-called zero-cord (lead) may be used. This can only be done on the basis of expert electrical installation. In many instances, it turns out to be better to use a special grounding connection with a sheet of copper merged in the ground water level. Note: The lightning rod should never be used, since high power energies should not penetrate into the interior of the house. When the water pipe is taken for grounding, it has to be assured that there excists a metallic connection to the earth (no plastic materials). The grounding should always be done by an electric expert.

23.6.2.

On top of the grounded metal mesh one should place a layer of insulating material, which must not be chargeable by friction. We would recommend a coco mat or a light rattan carpet. Under no circumstances should coverings out of plastic materials be used, since they tend to recharge thus spoiling the measurement results (see above).

23.6.3.

The utilization of "antistatic liquids" which prevent coverings of plastic material from being charged is to be recommended and should be done as a common practice. In addition, a carpet as flooring material is always recommendable.

The cheapest method to annihilate static electrical fields or avoid their formation is spraying water. Furthermore, there exist textile fabrics of various mixtures which cannot be charged. The same applies to carpet mats, which, however, are pretty expensive.

23.7.

Since it is the patient and not the instrument which is highly influenced by electric fields, in particular by low and high frequency alternating electric fields, one has to make sure that these fields do not form.

Since no generally binding advice can be given on that because of individual circumstances present, an expert in "biologically adequate building" should be consulted.

In any case, low frequency alternating fields may be spotted with the aid of an acoustic field detecting device made by *Kraiss & Friz,* Stuttgart. Fields, in particular, are disturbing measurements when they are inhomogenous, thus creating interferences. Such interferences have to be avoided, also in your sleeping room.

The *Kraiss & Friz Company* also supplies a field intensity measurement device in order to detect points of interferences in the high frequency range. This instrument, however, is rather expensive.

The author of this book can supply any instrument on demand, also on a leasing basis.

The *K+F-Diatherapuncteur* is the basis for all other EAV-instruments.

Therefore, the *K+F-Diatherapuncteur* shall be described in more detail, although, it is no longer being manufactured.

Description of the K+F-Diatherapuncteur

The *K+F-Diatherapuncteur* is composed of two parts independent of each other but housed in one casing and is supplied with one cord to the mains.

Diagnostic part

The one part of the "K+F-Diatherapuncteur" constitutes the diagnostic instrument consisting essentially of a so-called ohmic tube (valve) meter, or rather volt tube meter.

The diagram in Figure 1 shows an electron tube (triode), the anode current of which is measured by a measuring device to give the maximum reading at 3 mA. The cathode is situated over the resistance Rk at the negative pole possessing at the resistance R 1 a positive potential against the negative pole. The cathode resistance Rk is installed as a potentiometer and may supply any desired negative voltage before reaching the grid of the tube. The tube characteristic in Fig. 1, upper left corner, shows that at a certain negative voltage before the grid the anode current IA becomes 0, i.e., the tube is blocked. In order to decrease the sensitivity of the measuring device towards polarization currents, a displacement of the zero mark has been provided by considerably raising the negative voltage before the grid. A polarization voltage and thus a polarization current may result from a battery effect between the electrodes and sweat; for this, the various sizes of the electrodes are important. The grid (negative) is connected via the relay contacts of a relay shunt to the black banana plug, which in turn is inserted into the hand-electrode. The tip of the stylus (positive pole) is connected to a potentiometer (hand reel below the measurement instrument) which has to be turned so that the measurement instrument yields a maximum indicator deviation (100) after depressing the knob left to the hand reel, that is, after short circuiting the electrodes (this applies only to the tube meters).

The measuring voltage applied to the patient on the acupuncture point ranges between 135 to 2070 mV, that is, on an average 900 mV depending on the magnitude of the pseudo-resistance. The current passing through the body thus ranges between 11.25 to 5.50 micro amperes (see Fig. 2).

The diagnostic part of the instrument, at first sight, appears to be a device for measuring the resistance of the skin on the acupuncture point. The measurement instrument shows an indicator deviation of 50, that is, 50 per cent of the scale as long as the acupuncture point and the corresponding organ are free from pathologic disturbances. An ohmic resistance of approx. 100 kilo ohm (exactly 95 K ohm), which is connected to the two electrodes instead of the human body, likewise reaches an indicator deviation of 50 units. Apart from this, I was

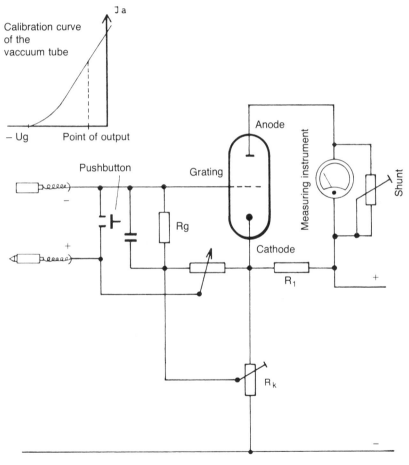

Fig. 1: Diagram of connections of the diagnostic part of the K+F-Diatherapuncteur apparatus.

able to evidence that a voltage of approx. 0.87 volt as opposed to the voltage in the instrument, also gives an indicator deviation of 50.

Fig. 2 shows the calibration curves of the diagnostic part of the "K+F-Dia-therapuncteur" instrument. An ohmic resistance of 27 kilo ohm gives an indicator deviation of 80, and 129 kilo ohm gives an indicator deviation of 40 per cent (solid curve). The corresponding voltages applied to the body range between 300 and 1090 mV (interrupted curve). Next to this are listed the calculated currents passing through the point of the body in that respective moment. Thus, the normal value of 50 is associated with 95 k ohm and 870 mV (approx. 1 volt).

Hypothesis for operating the diagnostic part of the instrument.

It is a known fact that acupuncture points exhibit different properties in comparison to their dermal environment, which can be checked by electrical measurement devices. Both the alternating current resistance and the direct current resistance of the acupuncture points are less than those of other "neutral" random points. The neutral points do not lie in the vicinity of established acupuncture points, nor do they lie in the vicinity of meridians. When locating the acupuncture points a precise knowlegde of the positions of the points is necessary. The acupuncture points, on the surface of the skin, exhibit optimal values within diameters of 2 to 3 mm.

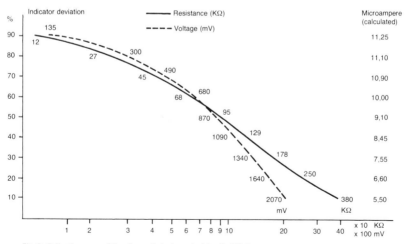

Fig. 2: Calibration curve of the diagnostic instrument of the K+F-Diatherapuncteur apparatus.

The acupuncture meridians have to be considered as energetic pathways, on which the acupuncture points are situated. With the aid of sensitive measurement devices these meridians can be checked on the living body. They are, in fact, a reality. A further proof for this was furnished by *Niboyet* and his co-workers when he fed electric direct current into a dermal area specimen to derive it from a different location, which could be done optimally only on dermal spots denoted as acupuncture points and which were combined by the so-called meridians. The individual meridians do not exist separately but are interrelated by secondary vessels. As long as there is bioelectric energy in the body, all meridians will be supplied more or less by bio-electric energy.

The acupuncture points may be regarded as battery like formations. A proof for this may be furnished in that a galvanometer of high ohmic resistance, whose poles are connected to one hand-electrode and one stylus-electrode respectively, shows a much higher reading on the acupuncture point than on a random point on the skin which is neither connected to a meridian nor situated in the vicinity of an acupuncture point.

The polarization current present between sweat and electrode is by far less than the bio-electric current, which may be derived from the acupuncture point.

Obviously, the body produces a potential in the organs to reach the acupuncture point via the meridians. The charge on the individual acupuncture point caused by the exactly definable current of our measurement device (see Fig. 2), creates a state of balance between the irritational potential and the body's potential, both of which are opposite to each other. The body processes the irritational current in the acupuncture point. The result of this reaction is the deviation of the indicator on the measurement scale denoting the corresponding situation of balance. The potential in a healthy body, therefore, impedes the intrusion of the irritational potenial into the body. The indicator of the measuring instrument remains on "50" and does not move, neither upwards nor downwards.

This gives us sufficient evidence to believe, in contrast to other allegations, that we are not dealing exclusively with a resistance measurement but rather with the reactive potential of the body's organs as opposed to a measurement current applied to the body, that is, to the organ meridian. This could be proved by a test in which the resistance of the body against the electric current, (measured between hand–hand) depending on the measuring current in a special array, could be established. As a result, the resistance of the person to be measured climbs from 0 volt upwards until reaching a maximum, from which it starts dropping again. The voltage for reaching this maximum varies individually ranging between 0.5 volts in elder people to 1.4 volts in younger test persons. This proves that up to a certain irritational voltage, that is, to the maximum value corresponding to the individual, the rising resistance of the person's body may impede the intrusion of the electrical current into the body within physiologic magnitudes. After trespassing this magnitude the body can no longer cope with the measuring voltage to result in a fatigued reaction as to the irritational current. It turned out, furthermore, that a repeated measurement taken immediately after the first test within the range of low voltage shows the resistance to be higher than in the first measurement. The body, therefore, is still in a state of "defence". The "every-thing-or-nothing law" in electro-physiology established, that the body can react only to a stimulus, which trespassed the stimulus threshold.

This may be expected to be true, when we are exclusively dealing with the central nervous system via reflex terminals and when the stimulus becomes visible, for example in the form of a contraction of the muscle. In our case, however, the stimulus is low-level (subliminal) to a large degree. The cerebro-spinal nervous system, therefore, can by no means be irritated. It is only the autonomic nervous system, which responds. In order to assure a useful differentiation of the measurement result, measuring current and measuring voltage have to remain within the confines of magnitudes allowing the organs to react adequately. When the stimulus is too little, that is, the measurement device is too sensitive, the organ will always be capable of counter-balancing the irritational current. In this case, we will not achieve any indicator drop. On the other hand, in applying a strong stimulus or a short circuit represented, for example, by a high calibre resistance measurement device of 8 to 10 kilo ohm's internal resistance, an indicator drop will always be present. Only the proper physiologic dimension of the irritational current will facilitate a state of balance between irritation and reaction in normotonic conditions of the body resulting in a stable indicator deviation.

When, according to the mathematical law, two magnitudes equal a third one, they also have to equal each other. This leads us to accept that the potential of an organ when charged by the diagnostic part of the K +F-Diatherapuncteur, lies in the magnitude of o. 87 volts, on the supposition of a physiologic condition present in the acupuncture point. The measurement reading should be = 50 (see also Fig. 2).

My theroy, that the acupuncture point supplies an electromotor force and can be regarded as a battery-like formation is in agreement with outlines of Prof. Kracmar, Vienna. The substitute diagram of connections he submitted in Bad Nauheim 1961 for the acupuncture point, namely the parallel connection of a resistance and a condenser, fully applies to a galvanic element (battery). This element, also, has an internal ohmic resistance depending on the magnitude of the electrodes and the concentration of the electrolyte and a capacitance factor. In the human body, in addition, the resistance and the capacitance vary in the course of time. Both magnitudes depend on the state of ionisation of the electrolyte, that is, the intercellular body liquids. The state of ionisation may change in varying concentration of the electrolyte (lack or surplus, blocs or difficulties of excretion) or because of additional stronger ionising electrolytes (toxins).

An equilibrium between stimulus and reaction will not be reached, when the response of the body to be examined is insufficient, such as in lack of energy. The indicator drop, characteristic of a lack of response of the organ related to the meridian to be examined, will always be present and always be reproducible. Also, the demand for an electrode of constant pressure will be seen in a different light, when one considers that it is not an ohmic resistance but a potential from the body, that is, an electro-motor force which is measured on the acupuncture point. The wetting of the electrode, i.e., the reduction of the resistance of the uppermost corium as well as a strong pressure on the acupuncture point are sufficient to connect the energy sources of the body with the electrode of the stylus and thus with the measuring instrument in which a possible incorrectness of the measurement must not exceed the usual ± 1.5 per cent when the point-electrode has been placed on the acupuncture point (approx. one scale unit in values ranging about 80).

It could be approved by many tests that the increase of the contact pressure applied by the point-electrode on the acupuncture point cannot keep the indicator from dropping in case of a pathologic condition on the acupuncture point. A proper measurement is always based on a precise location of the acupuncture point. A buzzer incorporated into the "K+F-Diatherapuncteur" makes the location of the point easier.

Professor *Kracmar,* Vienna, was asked by Dr. *Voll* to examine the problem of the pressure-constant electrode and he submitted the following report to us:

As I communicated to you, we have made an electrode of constant pressure in our workshop. I put this electrode to various tests on which I want to report. As an electrode we took the "little electrode" normally used by electro-acupuncturists. When this electrode was applied on various acupuncture points without using pressure, the instrument showed only a slight indicator deviation. The normal value of the indication (50 scale units) was reached only when pressure of the spring of approx. 1 kg (= 1000 pond) was exercised. Judging by the manner the tissue is compressed, this pressure of the spring appears to me as being of the same magnitude like the contact pressure of the electrode of inconstant pressure which I observed in tests of Dr. *Kollmer* and Dr. *Schramm.* In direct current measurement, therefore, used in EAV-diagnostics, the pressure of the electrode seems to have to be larger than in the alternating current measurement. In my tests carried out so far – which should be controlled by you or Dr. *Kollmer* jointly – the electrode of inconstant pressure appears to be suitable to render fault-free measurement results on the condition that it is placed on the measurement spot with equally strong pressure. The strength of the applied contact pressure depends on experience which could be simplified by marking the mobile bolt on the electrode developed by me.

Notwithstanding the above outlines, a stylus for constant pressure was made by the Kraiss & Friz Company, Stuttgart, following the recommendations of Prof.

Kracmar, Vienna, and may be supplied on request to anyone willing to do research on this field of electroacupuncture. Tests with this stylus revealed, that for proper measurements a contact pressure of the electrode of at least 500 to 600 grams is required. In a higher contact pressure applied by the electrode the indicator deviation on the diagnostic meter of the instrument changes only slightly until a pathologic pressure is reached which is stated by the patient to be very painful.

Remark: In the meantime, the above mentioned facts could be confirmed by tests using a double circle recording instrument: The contact pressure of the electrode of the stylus applied to the skin on the acupuncture point may be varied within limits, as mentioned, between 600 ponds to 1600 ponds, which results in no changes of the measurement value. A pressure-constant electrode of simple make for proper values requires measurements perpendicular to the surface of the skin, which may be difficult. When placing the measuring stylus obliquely, the cylinder applying the pressure has too much friction and thus falsifies the measurement result.

Note: Measurement techniques to-day facilitate to reach proper results in connection with complicated electronic gadgets as well as the above mentioned double circle recorder, even if the stylus is placed obliquely.

Finally, I should like to point out that there exist a great number of diagnostic electronic instruments, such as the various electro-cardiographs, electro-encephalographs, Rilling's instrument and others using the body's own electrical voltage for measurements. In addition, there are instruments by means of which one can take measurements of the skin resistance only, to draw diagnostic conclusions (*Croon's* apparatus).

Also, thermal irradiation, like ultra-red-irradiation, can be measured in its varying intensity emanated by the body (*Schwamm's* apparatus). I am not aware of any procedure, which by charging the acupuncture points using pure direct current in physiologic magnitudes, facilitates a functional diagnosis easy to differentiate like in electro-acupuncture.

What we measure, is the reaction of the organ in the acupuncture points caused by the irritational current of physiologic magnitude. This irritational current is in the order of 5.5 to 11.25 microamps with measurement readings between 10 to 90 on the meter scale depending on the organ potential which has to be overcome (2070 mV in an indicator deviation of 10, up to 135 mV in an indicator deviation of 90). The organ potential is directly proportional to the seeming ohmic resistance.

The therapy part of the instrument

The number of therapeutic electronic devices is admittedly very large, ranging from thermal lamps, ultra-violet lamps to apparatuses using medium frequencies between 50 and 100 hertz and even ultra-sound and ultra-shortwave instruments as well as x-ray and isotope instruments for therapy. All of these instruments use pure sinusoidal oscillations. In addition, there are instruments using the so-called Leduc's currents, that is, oscillations of rectangular shape. Furthermore, there are a number of other instruments used for research applying any kind of curve characteristic. But only one instrument is known using relaxation (kipp) oscillations of exactly defined shape as well as frequencies ranging between 0.8 to 10 hertz of equal or variable cycles, this being the therapeutic part of the *K+F-Diatherapuncteur* as well as the *Dermatron*.

The therapeutic part contains a generator for relaxation-oscillations with a gliding frequency adjustment between 0.8 to 10 hertz, which may either be turned on by hand or may be varied by a small electric motor or electronic device. What are relaxation-oscillations? A relaxation oscillation may be any oscillation not following a sinusoidal curve. Any kind of a weird oscillation, which includes relaxation oscillations may be split up by harmonics analysis into sinusoidal oscillations of varying frequencies and intensities. Conversely, one may build up any curve characteristic by summarizing sinusoidal oscillations of varying frequencies and intensities.

The shape of oscillations created in the *K+F-Diatherapuncteur* adapts closely to the oscillations received in the EKG. (Figure 3 shows the oscillograms of these oscillations.)

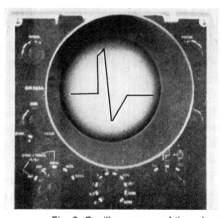 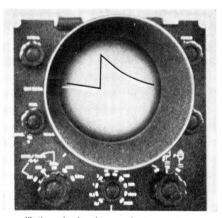

Fig. 3: Oscillogrammes of the relaxation oscillations in the therapy instrument.
Left: Alternating relaxation oscillations for "increasing" (Aufbau).
Right: Positive direct current relaxation oscillation used for "decreasing" (Abbau).

The curves shown on Fig. 3 representing alternating and direct current relaxation oscillations should rather be designated as "impulses", since a relatively rapid electric event is always followed by an interval which is mostly larger than the "impulse" itself. The impulse contains a high percentage of oscillations of very low frequencies. It is the basic oscillation which determines the frequency of the impulses. In addition, oscillations of low intensity up to the ultra short wave realm (between 80 and 100 megahertz) can be evidenced as being comparable to the harmonics of a tone (sound). The band width of the relaxation oscillations produced in the $K+F$-Diatherapuncteur, therefore, is very large. The interval following the impulse corresponds to the refractory time of the tissue in our body, which may range between 0.1 seconds for the heart muscle to 0.001 seconds for the sceleton muscle.

It turned out that in practical applications the relaxation oscillations produced in the "K+F-Diatherapuncteur" are very effective from a physiologic point of view since the interval between the impulses take care of the regeneration of the tissue(nervous potential)

Fig. 4 shows the connection diagram of the therapeutic instrument: An oscillation generator and a successive amplifier, formed simultaneously as an impulse corrector. The alternating relaxation oscillations produced by the instrument may be applied to the body by means of the electrodes via a potentiometer for in-

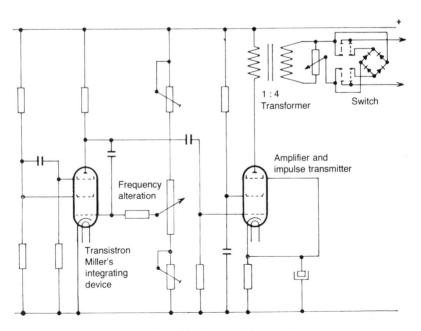

Fig. 4: Diagram of connections of the therapeutic instrument.

tensity control or, alternatively after rectification, as direct current relaxation oscillations. Both curve characteristics change their intensity as per unit of time. This makes possible that a direct current relaxation oscillation may increase the body's charge using larger intensity, in other words, increasing the conductance value or, biologically speaking, removing a bloc (*Oltrogge*).

This is in contrast to our usual directions for operating the instrument with respect to direct current relaxation oscillations, when only the least intensity should be applied.

The explanation for this may be that a direct current relaxation oscillation of major intensity constitutes a physiologic stimulus, which is answered in the body by an increase of the energy flow. The difference between the direct current relaxation oscillation of major intensity and the alternating relaxation oscillation of large intensity is the more intensive effect of the latter on the sensitive nervous system, in that the peaks of intensity exercise an additional irritation. The area comprised by the curve and the zero line is an expression for the amount of energy supplied to the body in the form of the impulse. Fig. 3 clearly shows that the direct current relaxation oscillation yields an amount of energy many times larger than that of the alternating relaxation oscillation. One can imagine that only the peak voltages penetrate the fatty tissue around the sensitive nerves thus causing an irritation and it is clear that the magnitude of the amplitude of the direct current relaxation oscillation need not be that high for the same amount of energy to be released. In special cases, therefore, one can apply direct current relaxation oscillations of major energy whose peak voltages do not exceed the irritation threshold and whose electric effects (tingling) will not be felt as being painful.

In copy No. 4/1975 of the American Journal of Acupuncture in a paper by Dr. Voll on "Twenty years of Acupuncture therapy using low frequency current pulses" on seven pages the indications of the individual frequencies are described. This paper is also included in the special copy of the American Journal of Acupuncture entitled "Electro-acupuncture according to Voll" in 1978. This special copy contains the five papers of Dr. Voll published previously by the American Journal of Acupuncture. The indications of the frequencies are listed on this copy on pages 29 to 35.

I should like to stress once more that in using current for the treatment of the patient no discomfort must be present on the part of the patient. As soon as the cerebro-spinal nervous system gets irritated by the electric currents we reach the opposite of our desired effects in the body. Instead of reaching spasmolysis we may come across vehement spasms. This may also be illustrated by the occurrance of tetany in high power accidences.

The application of the *K+F-Diatherapuncteur* requires the knowledge of the implications of classical acupuncture. The instrument makes the location of the topographic positions of the points easy.

The K+F-Diatherapuncteur is a valuable aid in the daily practice and one will find this rewarding when one can master the instrument rather than the other way around. As to additional remarks concerning the application of positive or negative direct current impulses and their intensity, Dr. Voll stresses the following:

1. When, in sensitive persons, the application of the alternating current impulses of strong intensity is causing discomfort the positive direct current impulse of major intensity should be used. A voltage between the peak and the zero line of the direct current impulse is much lower than the voltage between peak to peak of the alternating current impulse.

2. The increase (charging) of the body's potential by means of direct current positive impulses whith major current intensity may, in exceptional cases, lead to a strong drop of the conductance values and thus to collapse-like situations (oral report by Dr. Ehmann). This is why these current impulses should be applied only when controlling the newly established conductance value in regular time intervals using the "automatic" switch.

3. The alternating current impulse, in contrast to the negative direct current impulse (pseudo charging), is capable of recharging the energetic reservoirs of our body situated on the course of the wonder meridians. This effect may last longer.

4. In order to achieve a quicker recharging up to conductance values of more than 80 in energetic low voltages one starts by using the negative direct current impulses (pseudo charging) for 1/2 minute, to switch over subsequently to the alternating current impulses. This assures the recharging of the energetic reservoirs for a longer period of time.

Appendix

Locations of the acupuncture points on the terminal parts of the extremities

Medial   Lateral

YIN: negative; female; mother like; passive; wet; cold; dark; receptive; mystical; concealing; shade; water;

YANG: positive; male; father like; active; dry; warm; light; creative; constant; beaming; sun; fire;

	I	II	III	IV	V	
Hand	Lu.	LI.	Cir.S.	End.	He. / SI.	
						YIN-points
						YANG-points
	Ly.	Ner.	All.	■		Particular-points
				■		Degeneration-points
Foot	r. Pa. / l. Sp. / Li.	St.	Skin	Gbl.	Ky. / UB.	
						YIN-points
						YANG-points
		artic.	fibr.	fatty		Particular-points
						Degeneration-points

The black square marks the position of the parenchymal and epithelial degeneration vessel (see Illustrated Vol. II, Fig. 31).

Initial and terminal parts of the Yang and Yin meridians

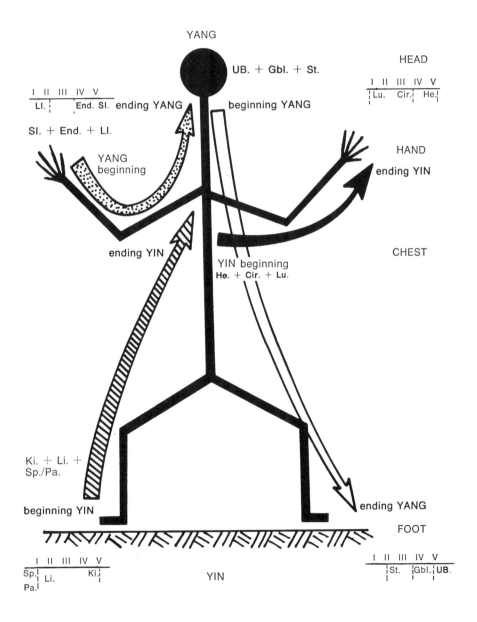

YANG

UB. + Gbl. + St.

HEAD

I II III IV V
Lu.   Cir. He.

I II III IV V
LI.   End. SI. ending YANG

beginning YANG

SI. + End. + LI.

YANG
beginning

HAND

ending YIN

ending YIN

YIN beginning
He. + Cir. + Lu.

CHEST

Ki. + Li. +
Sp./Pa.

ending YANG

beginning YIN

FOOT

I II III IV V
Sp.   Ki.
Li.
Pa.

YIN

I II III IV V
St.   Gbl. UB.

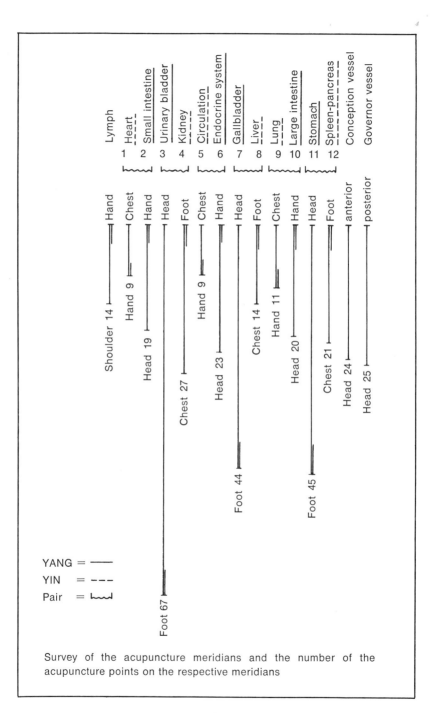

Survey of the acupuncture meridians and the number of the acupuncture points on the respective meridians

YANG = ———
YIN = – – –
Pair = ᴸᴡᴡᴶ

The organ clock for maximum times in the circadian system of the circulation of energy

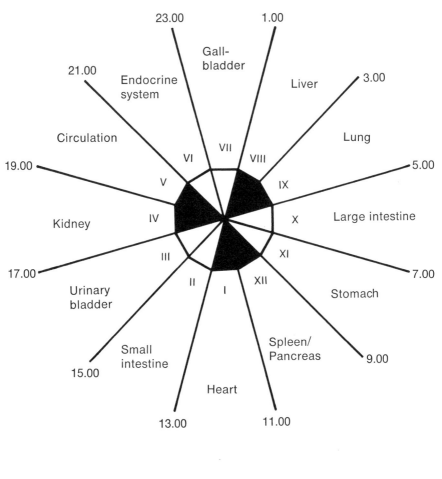

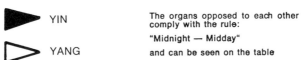

YIN

YANG

The organs opposed to each other comply with the rule:

"Midnight — Midday"

and can be seen on the table

Interrelations of the organs

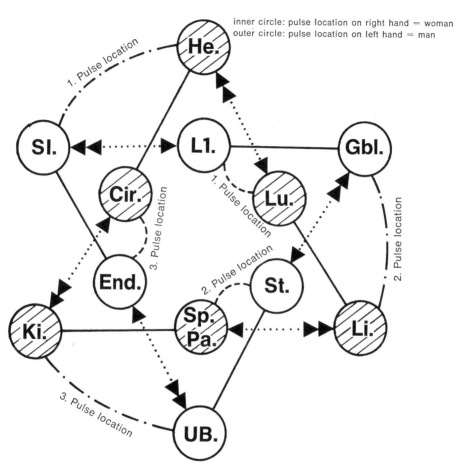

inner circle: pulse location on right hand = woman
outer circle: pulse location on left hand = man

1. Pulse location

He.

Sl.

Ll.

Gbl.

Cir.

Lu.

3. Pulse location

1. Pulse location

2. Pulse location

End.

St.

2. Pulse location

Ki.

Sp. Pa.

Li.

3. Pulse location

UB.

Law of the parallel pulse relations

1. ·······▶ Relations MAN—WOMAN (traditional acupuncture)
2. ◀ ◀ ····· Relations RIGHT—LEFT pulse location
3. ———— Law of crossed relations of pulse locations
  (see page 220)

 YIN: deep pulse
location

 YANG: superficial pulse
location

Therapeutic currents fed into the acupuncture points

curve characteristic	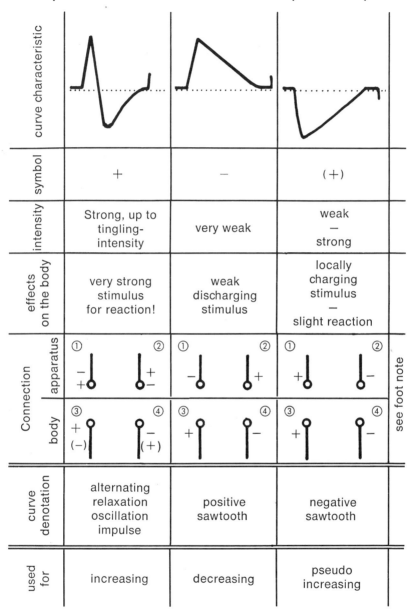		
symbol	+	−	(+)
intensity	Strong, up to tingling-intensity	very weak	weak − strong
effects on the body	very strong stimulus for reaction!	weak discharging stimulus	locally charging stimulus − slight reaction
Connection — apparatus / body	① −⊥+● ② +⊥●− ③ +⊥(−)● ④ −⊥●(+)	① −⊥● ② +⊥●+ ③ +⊥● ④ −⊥●	① +⊥● ② −⊥●− ③ +⊥● ④ −⊥●
curve denotation	alternating relaxation oscillation impulse	positive sawtooth	negative sawtooth
used for	increasing	decreasing	pseudo increasing

① corresponds to the hand-electrode   ③ corresponds to the hand of the
② corresponds to the stylus-electrode   patient
                                   ④ corresponds to the acupuncture
                                   point

Remarks regarding the figure: Therapy currents applied on the acupuncture point.

Under item 7.1.1. I have tried to outline that the human body is capable of releasing an electric charge on the acupuncture points many times higher than the polarization voltage of the surrounding skin. It could be established that the interior of the body via the sweat glands of the hand together with the hand electrodes form a positive potential, while the stylus on the acupuncture point yields a negative potential. To repeat some physical terminology:

a) Negative electricity is present, when the object to be measured exhibits a surplus of electrons, that is the carriers of electric energy.

b) Positive electricity exhibits a lack of electrons.

c) "Polarization" denotes the formation of a field (electromotor force) by means of ionization in an electrolyte such as sweat, which can be lead off by electrodes of equal composition and can be made measurable.

d) The term of "polarity" refers to the outlines under a) and b) and is denoted by plus (+) and minus (−).

From these considerations it is obvious that apart from warmth and perspiration the human body also gets rid of bio electric energy in the form of negative electrons to balance the surplus created by the processing of nutrition. When the discharge of electrons becomes too high in a conducting medium, such as smog, i.e., higher than the production of bio-electric energy in the body, the body becomes impoverished, that is, hypo-energetic. On the other hand, when clothes which are charged negatively impede the flow of electrons (equal poles repel each other), this concentration of energy for a short time is felt to be pleasant; after a certain lapse of time, however, discharge of energy may cause discomfortable side-effects.

Considering all this, the schematic diagramm of current flow in the body and the instrument may be explained as follows:

a) The human body exhibits on the acupuncture point a (relatively speaking) negative potential and in the body itself a positive potential.

b) Figuratively, we may visualize the acupuncture point as being a small accumulator which is fed by bio-electric energy from the inside of the body.

c) When this litte accumulator is discharged by placing a charge of opposite poles on it, an energy deficit would result on this charged spot. Since the body does not tolerate such a deficit, a correspondig amount of bio-electric energy is supplied immediately to achieve what has been requested by Voll: The transformation of a static condition into a dynamic one, or in other words: the bio-electric energy starts flowing again. This is essentially what happens in the "positive direct current relaxation oscillation" for decreasing and in the "alternating relaxation oscillation" increasing the charge. In the first case, only a weak stimulus is present with a corresponding reaction. There are no reactions of the sensitive nervous system but only on the part of the autonomic nervous system. The stimulus of the alternating relaxation oscillation is strong in that the energy can be felt by a tingling sensation involving the sensitive nerves. The reaction, therefore, also is strong and lasting.

For many years we have achieved good results using these two curve characteristics. One day somebody suggested to reverse the "sawtooth", which can better be accomplished technically, and to apply "negative direct current relaxation oscilations" to the body. It seemed at first sight as if the charging effect took place more quickly. An examination revealed, however, that the charging effect.

was only of short duration. One may visualize this process in that the "accumulator" of the acupuncture point gets charged locally, thus rendering its functional area conductible after the application of relatively low energy. However, the desired effect of the flow of bio-electric energy is not reached to any major extent. Only when applying larger amounts of energy by means of alternating relaxation oscillations and over a longer period of time, a longer lasting charging effect will result since energetic reservoirs are also recharged this way. The otherwise energetically impoverished reservoirs are responsible for the sufficient energetic supply, in particular in situations of emergency.

Abbreviations for the following tables

AP. = Acupuncture point with its meridian
MP. = Measurement point
End. = Triple warmer – endocrine meridian
GV. = Governor vessel
CV. = Conception vessel
Ly. = Lymph vessel
D   = right
S   = left

Index of abbreviations:
l   = left
r   = right
Ly. = Lymph
Ci. = Circulation
Al. = Allergy
End. = 3-W = 3-Warmer (Endocrine)
Gov. = Governor
Con. = Conception
Gbl. = Gallbladder
Li. = Liver
He. = Heart
Ki. = Kidney
UB. = Urinary bladder
St. = Stomach
Lu. = Lung
Sp. = Spleen
Pa. = Pancreas
LI. = Large intestine
SI. = Small intestine

Fig. 1 MP.

101	19. Sl.	External ear
102	9. St.	Parathyroid
103*	15. Sl.	Pituitary gland
	16. End.	
	21. Gbl.	
104	11. St.	Thymus
105	15 Ll.	Shoulder-arm joint 1st Mp.
106	11 Ll.	Elbow joint 3rd MP.
107	3 Ci.	Elbow joint 2nd MP.
108	7. Lu.	Arteries of the upper extremities
109	8. Lu.	Veins of the upper extremities
+613		
110	33. Gbl.	Joints of the lower extremities
111	35. St.	Knee joint 2nd MP.
112	34. Gbl.	Muscles of the lower extremities
113	9. Sp.Pa.	Lymph vessels of the lower extremities
114	8. Sp.Pa.	Urogenital diaphragm
115	7. Sp.Pa.	Pelvic diaphragm
116	41. St.	Ankle joint 2nd MP.
117	62. UB.	Posterior talocalcaneal joint
118	2. Ci.	Shoulder-arm joint 2nd MP.
119	10. St.	Thyroid
120	10a. St.	Vagus nerve
121	30. St.	Hip joint 1st MP.
122	11a. Sp.Pa.	Hip joint 2nd MP.
123*	12. Li.	Ovary
	11. Sp.Pa.	Testis
	31. St.	
124	32. St.	Arteries of the lower extremities
125	33. St.	Abdominal veins
126	10. Sp.Pa.	Pelvic veins
127	7. Li.	Veins of the lower extremities
128	8. Li.	Knee joint 1st MP.
129*	8. Ki.	Blood
	6. Sp.Pa.	Hemorrhage
	5. Li.	
130	3. Ki.	Pyelo-renal region of the kidney
+516		
131	6. Ki.	Anus + Rectum
+517		
132	2. Ki.	Pyelo-renal region of the kidney
+519		
133	5. Sp.Pa.	Ankle joint

** points of intersections of three meridians
** 10a. Stomach

Anterior Aspect of the Body

Measurement points in Electro-acupuncture according to Voll

101	19. SI.	118	2. Ci.
102	9. St.	119	10. St.
103*	+	120	10a. St.
104	11. St.	121	30. St.
105	15 LI.	122	11a.St.
106	11 LI.	123*	+
107	3 Ci.	124	32. St.
108	7. Lu.	125	33. St.
109	8. Lu.	126	10. Sp. Pa.
110	33. Gbl.	127	7. Li.
111	35. St.	128	8. Li.
112	34. Gbl.	129*	+
113	9. Sp. Pa.	130	3. Ki.
114	8. Sp. Pa.	131	6. Ki.
115	7. Sp. Pa.	132	2. Ki.
116	41. St.	133	5. Sp. Pa.
117	62. UB.		

1

* points of intersections of three meridians
** 10a. Stomach

Fig. 2 MP.

201	21. End.	Anterior portion of the eye
202	1. Gbl.	Posterior portion of the eye
203	5. St.	Maxillary sinus
204	20. End.	Hypothalamus
205	23. End.	Upper jaw joint
206	2. St.	Lower jaw joint
207	25. Gov.	Upper teeth
208	7. St.r	Upper teeth, right
208	7. St.l	Upper teeth, left
209	8a St.	Submandibular gland
210	8. St.r	Lower teeth, right
210	8. St.l	Lower teeth, left
211	23a Con.	Tongue
212	23a Gov.	Cavity of the nose
213	2. UB.	Frontal sinus
214	*	Sphenoidal sinus
215	20. Ll.	Ethmoid cells
216	3a St.	Lingual tonsil
217	3. St.	Parotid gland
218	24. Con.	Upper teeth
219	23a Con.	Pharyngeal tonsil
220 +608	18. Ll.	Tubal tonsil
221	17. Ll.	Laryngeal tonsil

* situated on the secondary vessel between 20. Ll. to 1. UB.

Measurement Points in Electro-acupuncture according to Voll

212	23a Gov.
213	2. UB.
214 *	
215	20. LI.
216	3a St.
217	3. St.
208	7. St.l
210	8a St.l
218	24. Con.
220	18. LI.
221	17. LI.
219	23a Con.

201	21. End.
202	1. Gbl.
203	5. St.
204	20. End.
205	23. End.
206	2. St.
207	25. Gov.
208	7. St.r
209	8a St.r
210	8. St.r
211	23a Con.

2

* situated on the secondary vessel between 20. LI. to 1. UB.

111

Fig. 3 MP.

301	19. End.	Meninges
302	18. End.	Internal ear
303	17. End.	Middle ear
304	20. Gbl.	Sympathetic nerve
305	14. End.	Acromioclavicular joint
306	10. Sl.	Shoulder-arm joint
307	9. Sl.	Muscles of the upper extremities
308	8. Sl.	Elbow joint 1st MP.
309	7. Sl.	Nerves of the upper extremities
310	49a UB.	Epididymis – Ostium abdominale tubae
311	49b UB.	Ductus deferens – Ampulla tubae uterinae
312	49c UB.	Vesicula seminalis – Uterus pars interstitial. tubae uterinae
313	50. UB.	Prostate Uterus
314	51. UB.	Penis Vagina
315	54. UB.	Knee joint
316	39. Gbl.	Bone marrow
317	60. UB.	Nerves of the lower extremities
318	19. Gov.	Little brain
319	8. UB.	Epiphysis
320	17. Gov.	Corpora lamina quadrigemina
321	9. UB.	Pons Varoli
322	15. End.	Joints of the upper extremities
323	10. UB.	Medulla oblongata
324	13. Gov.	Medulla spinalis
325	11. UB.	Vertebral spine
326	12. UB.	Osseous system
327	17. UB.	Diaphragm
328	22. UB.	Adrenal gland
329	29. Gbl.	Hip joint 3rd MP.
330	29. UB.	Sacroiliacal joint
331	50a UB.	Seminal hillock Parameterium
332	51a UB.	Posterior portion of the urethra
333	52. UB.	Anterior portion of the urethra

End. = 3-W.

Posterior Aspect of the Body

Measurement Points in Electro-acupuncture according to Voll.

301	19.End.	318	19. Gov.
302	18.End.	319	8. UB.
303	17.End.	320	17. Gov.
304	20. Gbl.	321	9. UB.
305	14.End.	322	15.End.
306	10. SI.	323	10. UB.
307	9. SI.	324	13. Gov.
308	8. SI.	325	11. UB.
309	7. SI.	326	12. UB.
310	49a UB.	327	17. UB.
311	49b UB.	328	22. UB.
312	49c UB.	329	29. Gbl.
313	50. UB.	330	29. UB.
314	51. UB.	331	50a UB.
315	54. UB.	332	51a UB.
316	39. Gbl.	333	52. UB.
317	60. UB.		

3

Fig. 4 MP.

401	5. Sl.	Wrist joint
402	4. End.	Metacarpal joint
403	3. End.	Endocrinum (Hypophysis, Epiphysis)
404	4. Sl.r	Horizontal upper portion of the duodenum
404	4. Sl.l	Ascending portion of the duodenum
405	2. End.	Endocrinum (thyroid, thymus, parathyroid)
406	3. Sl.r	Descending portion of the duodenum
406	3. Sl.l	Flexura duodeno-jejunalis
407	2. Sl.r	Horizontal lower portion of the duodenum
407	2. Sl.l	Jejunum
408	1a Sl.r	Peritoneum of the duodenum
408	1a Sl.l	Peritoneum of the intestines
409	1. Sl.r	Terminal ileum
409	1. Sl.l	Ileum
410	9. He.r	Endocardium of the right ventricle
+622		Valve of the truncus pulmonalis
410	9. He.l	Endocardium of the left ventricle
+622		Aortic valve
411	1. End.	Endocrinium (Testis, Suprarenalis)
412	5. Ll.	Wrist joint
413	4a Ll.r	Appendix + ileo-coecal lymph nodes
413	4a Ll.l	Mesenteric lymph nodes
414	4. Ll.r	Coecum
414	4. Ll.l	Left-sided colon transversum
415	3. Al.	Allergy (Head, Face)
416	3. Ll.r	Colon ascendens
416	3. Ll.l	Flexura coli sinistra
417	2. Al.	Allergy (Upper extremities chest)
418	2. Ll.r	Flexura coli dextra
418	2. Ll.l	Colon descendens
419	11. Lu.	Lung, parenchyma and alveoli
+611		
420	1a Ll.	Peritoneum of the colon
421	1. Al.	Allergy (abdomen, lower extremities)
422	1. Ll.r	Right-sided colon transversum
422	1. Ll.l	Sigmoid
423	9. Ci.	Arteries
+612		

Dorsum of the right Hand
Measurement Points in Electro-acupuncture according to Voll

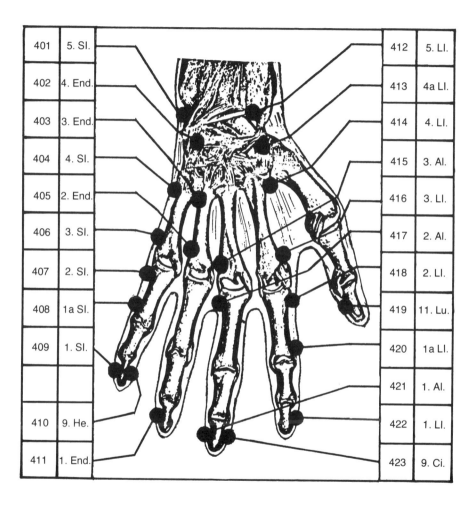

401	5. Sl.
402	4. End.
403	3. End.
404	4. Sl.
405	2. End.
406	3. Sl.
407	2. Sl.
408	1a Sl.
409	1. Sl.
410	9. He.
411	1. End.

412	5. Ll.
413	4a Ll.
414	4. Ll.
415	3. Al.
416	3. Ll.
417	2. Al.
418	2. Ll.
419	11. Lu.
420	1a Ll.
421	1. Al.
422	1. Ll.
423	9. Ci.

4

Fig. 5 MP.

501	39a Gbl.	Ankle joint
502	64. UB.	Ductus defer. Epididymis, Tuba uterina
503	41. Gbl.r	Ductuli biliferi dextri, Duct. hepatic. dextra
503	41. Gbl.l	Ductuli biliferi sinistri
504	3. Skin	Skin (Frace, Head)
505	65. UB.	Urinary Bladder
		Urethra anter. et poster., Vesicula et Colliculus
		seminalis, Prostate, Parametrium, Uterus, Pars
		interstitialis tubae uterinae, Penis, Vagina
506	42. Gbl.r	Body of the gallbladder
506	42. Gbl.l	Ductus hepaticus sinistra
507	1a Ki.	Ureter, abdominal portion
508	66. UB.	Trigonum vesicae
509	43. Gbl.	Ductus cysticus
510	2. Skin	Skin (chest, neck, nape, upper extremities)
511	67. UB.	Body of the urinary bladder
512	1. Ki.	Renal pelvis
513	44. Gbl.	Choledochal duct
513	44. Gbl.	Common hepatic duct
514	1. Skin	Skin (abdomen, back, small of the back, lower extremities)
515	45. St.r	Pylorus
515	45. St.l	Body of the stomach, left portion
516 +130	3. Ki.	Pyelorenal region of the kidney
517	6. Ki.	Rectum + Anus
518	4. Li.	Talocalcaneonavicular joint
519 +132	2. Ki.	Pyelorenal region of the kidney
520	42. St.	Upper portion of the esophagus
521	3. Li.	Capsula fibrosa regio periportalis of the liver
522	4. Pa.r	Pancreas, lipase formation
522	4. Sp.l	RES
523	43. St.r	Body of the stomach, right ascending portion
523	43. St.l	Cardia
524	3. Pa.r	Pancreas, amylase, insulin formation
524	3. Sp.l	Red pulp of the spleen
525	44. St.r	Antrum pyloricum of the stomach
525	44. St.l	Fundus of the stomach
526	2. Li.	Lobuli hepatici
527	2. Pa.r	Pancreas, nuclease formation
527	2. Sp.l	White pulp of the spleen
528	44a St.l	Peritoneum of the stomach, left portion
529	1. Li.	Central veins of the liver
530	1. Pa.r	Pancreas, protease formation
530	1. Sp.l	White pulp of the spleen

Dorsum of the right foot
Measurement Points in Electro-acupuncture according to Voll

501	39a Gbl.	516	3. Ki.
502	64. UB.	517	6. Ki.
503	41. Gbl.	518	4. Li.
504	3. Skin	519	2. Ki.
505	65. Gbl.	520	42. St.
506	42. Gbl.	521	3. Li.
507	1a Ki.	522	4. Sp. Pa.
508	66. UB.	523	43. St.
509	43. Gbl.	524	3. Sp. Pa.
510	2. Skin	525	44. St.
511	67. UB.	526	2. Li.
512	1. Ki.	527	2. Sp. Pa.
513	44. Gbl.	528	44a St.
514	1. Skin	529	1. Li.
515	45. St.	530	1. Sp. Pa

5

Fig. 6 MP.

601	6. Ly.	Lymph vessels of the upper extremities
602	5. Ly.	Lymph vessels of the heart and pericardium
603	8b Lu.	Larynx
604	4. Ly.	Lymph vessels of the lymph nodes of the lung and pleura + tracheobroncho-pulmonal and mediastinal lymph nodes
605	3. Ly.	Lymph vessels of the frontal, maxillary, shpenoid ethmoid sinus
606	10. Lu.	Bronchi
607	2. Ly.	Lymph vessels of the lymph nodes of the teeth, upper and lower jaw
608 +220	1a Ly.	Lymph vessels of the tubal tonsil
609	10a Lu.	Pleura
610	1. Ly.	Lymph vessel of the palatine tonsil
611 +419	11. Lu.	Lung parenchyma and alveoli
612	9. Ci.	Arteries
613 +109	8. Lu.	Veins of the upper extremities
614	8a Lu.	Pharynx
615	6. He.r	Heart muscle, right
615	6. He.l	Heart muscle, left
616	7. Ci.	Coronary arteries
617	9. Lu.	Trachea
618	7. He.	Atrioventricular fascicle
619	8. He.r	Endocardium, tricuspid valve of the right vestibule
619	8. He.l	Endocardium, mitral valve of the left vestibule
620	8. Ci.	Veins
612	8a He.r	Right pericardium
621	8a He.l	Left pericardium
622 +410	9. He.r	Endocardium, valve of the truncus pulmonalis of the right ventricle
622 +410	9. He.l	Endocardium, aortic valve of the left ventricle

Palm of the right Hand
on the dorsal side

Measurement Points in Electro-acupuncture according to Voll.

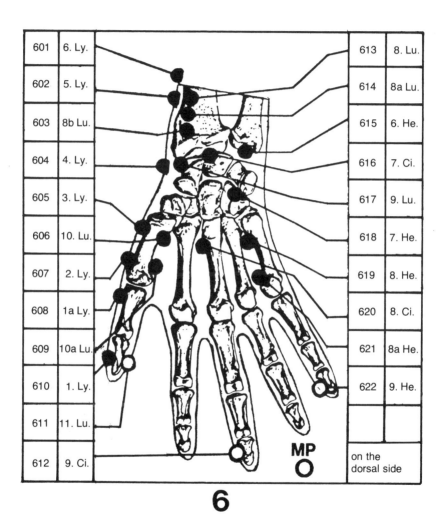

601	6. Ly.		613	8. Lu.
602	5. Ly.		614	8a Lu.
603	8b Lu.		615	6. He.
604	4. Ly.		616	7. Ci.
605	3. Ly.		617	9. Lu.
606	10. Lu.		618	7. He.
607	2. Ly.		619	8. He.
608	1a Ly.		620	8. Ci.
609	10a Lu.		621	8a He.
610	1. Ly.		622	9. He.
611	11. Lu.			
612	9. Ci.	MP ⭕	on the dorsal side	

6

Part II

Interpretation of the Rules of the Energy Exchange in Acupuncture

Introduction

For more than 23 years I have dealt with acupuncture many thousand years old. I am always surprised about the great experience contained in this method. To carry out acupuncture the acupuncterist is suited by rules and methods of treatment the may employ in therapy whenever a weak organ cannot be tonified via the common points. In this case he would take advantage of the rule of mother and son.

The doctor active in preventive medicine may use the rules of husband-and-housewife, as well as midnight-midday to treat the endangered organs simultaneous when an organ is diseased. The rule of the simultaneous treatment of a corresponding organ in a diseased organ is a further preventive and therapeutic law.

The energy present in the body has a circulation following the acupuncture teachings, i.e., the organs and their meridians are flooded in a certain sequence by this flowing energy. These maximum times of the organs are of physiologic and pathologic significance to man. Pathologic disturbances or pains occuring at certain times may serve as diagnostic hints as to the initial time of a disturbance. Thus, I considered it my task to discourse in detail in the following chapters the significance of these acupuncture rules for the use in the doctor's office. In addition to many examples I have given case reports in order to prove the correctness of these rules, which could also be supported by electro-acupuncture diagnosis and therapy. May these outlines convince the novice in acupuncture that it pays to deal with acupuncture and to use it as an adjunct in the daily practice. Disturbances and complaints filed in the anamnesis should always make reference to the time of the occurrance. This request may add to the evaluation of the anamnesis, in that the consideration of a maximum time already may serve as an early diagnosis for a functional disturbance of an organ.

Plochingen, June 1979   *Dr. med. Reinhold Voll*

Founder of Elektro-acupuncture and
Honorary President of the International Medical Association for
Electro-acupuncture according to Voll.

Maximum times (the organ clock).

Within the cycle of 24 hours the twelve large organs of the body are flooded each by the maximum energy of the body for two hours. Note, that the Chinese hour comprises two hours of our time measure According to the old acupuncture teaching, there exists a circulation of energy in the body. This energy, in succession, flows through the organs: heart, small intestine, urinary bladder, kidney, circulation, triple-warmer, (endocrine glands), gallbladder, liver, lung, large intestine, stomach, spleen pancreas – to return to the heart. The maximum times constitute a bio-rhythm.

The maximum times for each organ respectively are:

> Heart 11 a.m. to 1 p.m.
> Small intestine 1 to 3 p.m.
> Urinary bladder 3 to 5 p.m.
> Kidney 5 to 7 p.m.
> Circulation 7 to 9 p.m.
> Triple-warmer 9 to 11 p.m.
> Gallbladder 11 p.m. to 1 a.m.
> Liver 1 to 3 a.m.
> Lung 3 to 5 a.m.
> Large intestine 5 to 7 a.m.
> Stomach 7 to 9 a.m.
> Spleen-pancreas 9 to 11 a.m.

These maximum times are stated differently by a number of acupuncturists. *Bischko,* Vienna, in his book: "Introduction to Acupuncture" states the maximum times one hour later. *Chamfrault,* France, states the maximum times to be two hours earlier. Other authors like *Soulié de Morant, de la Fuye, Niboyet, Manaka,* Japan, and *Mann,* England, in their publications state the maximum times to be in accordance with my own experiences. On comparing the physiologic habits of men with the maximum times and on studying the occurrence of pain in the maximum times as hints to the etiology of diseases, one will be able to confirm the existence of maximum times as stated.

Which is the significance of the maximum times, physiologically speaking?

In its maximum time in the morning between 7 and 9 the stomach is in its highest function. During this time, the stomach is able to cope with a larger amount of nutrition than in other times of the day. Thus, the proverb proves the correctness of the maximum time of the stomach by stating: "In the morning you should eat like a rich man and in the evening you should eat like a beggar". During the maximum time of the stomach the uptake of alcohol occurs most rapidly, in other words alcoholemia occurs very quickly, while it is retarded in the minimum time of the stomach between 19 and 21. These results have been established by *Reinberg* and others in France in studies in chronobiology and chronopharmacology, as reported by Dr. *Bach* jun., Straßburg.

Stomach complaints outside the maximum time are due to mistakes in the diet, such as the intake of coffee, smoking, drinking of white wine or champagne etc. In this connection the following case report may be of interest:

A female patient complains about stomach pains each morning after rising up. These pains are also present in the evening when going to bed. The examination on the stomach points revealed no reason for these complaints, however, the measurement points for the plexus coeliacus = 44c. Stomach right and left exhibited large indicator drops. Medication testing using Mentha piperita D 6 for both coeliac plexus measurement points achieved the balancing down to 50. Thus, the reason for this disturbance could be verified to be peppermint in the tooth paste. From then on, the patient switched to tooth paste containing no peppermint, which is hard to obtain since most tooth pastes do contain peppermint or menthol. After this change, there have been no more stomach pains.

The spleen-pancreas has its maximum time at 9 to 11 in the morning. According to the old acupuncture teaching, the spleen-pancreas system in addition to its bodily functions has an influence on the mental action of our body, that is, on the mental activity and the capability to learn, likewise on our imagination and capability to concentrate. In short, the spleen-pancreas function is very important for our mental activity and productivity. This is why the maximum time of the spleen-pancreas between 9 and 11 is best for performing mental efforts, for example when learning a difficult subject which requires imaginative powers. The maximum time of the heart between 11 and 13 is the prerequisite for being able to digest larger amounts of food during the noon-time, this is when an increased blood circulation in the digestive organs is assured with the other parts of the body, like muscles and the brain, being equally supplied.

The maximum time of the small intestine is between 13 and 15. In acupuncture the duodenum is part of the small intestine. The small intestine has to break down the pre-digested nutritional agents by turning them into the smallest components of the intermediary metabolism, thus creating energy.

Pains in the upper abdomen between 13 and 15 are mostly due to pains in the duodenum originating either in the upper horizontal part due to a duodenal ulcer on the right side or in the ascending part of the duodenum on the left side. There exist isolated inflammatory processes of the ascending part of the duodenum when a frequent and spasmodic release of serotonin will occur. In this case, the pains chiefly located on the left side of the upper abdomen, are often mistaken for stomach complaints. Pains during this time occurring in the right lower abdomen originate in the terminal ileum as a first indication of an ileitis terminalis, i.e., Crohn's disease.

In acupuncture the small intestine is very closely related to the central and the peripheral nervous system, which is accounted for by successfully needling the small intestine points in diseases of the nervous system. For physiologic reasons one should not do any additional muscular work in the maximum time of the small intestine between 13 and 15, since this would cause a shift of blood supply into the muscular tissue and a deficiency of blood supply for the digestive functions of the small intestine, resulting in turn in an insufficient and incomplete fermentation of the ingested material. However, due to the working hours of man today, the small intestine is being damaged daily causing both insufficient fermentation on the part of the digestive glands and lack of resistivity of our central and peripheral nervous system. For men living in bio-rhythm it is indispensable to have a rest after the midday meal. In the southern regions, in the Mediterranean, people usually take a break after the midday meal, the more so, since the hot temperature during the noon hours forces them to slow down their work. This is equal to a forced biologic rest during this time.

The maximum time of the urinary bladder is between 15 and 17. A healthy person discharges most of his urine during this time of the day.

The maximum time of the kidney is between 17 and 19. Physiologically speaking, this accounts for the habit of having the five-o-clock-tea during this time which concides with the beginning of the maximum time of the kidneys to stimulate their functions by drinking black tea.

The maximum time of circulation between 19 and 21 does not relate to an organ but rather to a functional system, that is, the arterial and venous system of our body.

In the maximum time of the endocrine system between 21 and 23 the endocrine glands, responsible for the energy production in our body, are flooded. Particular physiologic hints cannot be given for this system, nor for the maximum time of the gallbladder, the liver, and lung.

As to the maximum time of the large intestine, it should be noted that a healthy large intestine will discharge stools during the time between 5 and 7.

What is the significance of the maximum times as to the pathologic complaints in the body?

When an organic function becomes insufficient, the maximum time will produce certain pathologic symptoms in various manifestations.

a) Pains in various manifestations, such as blunt, stinging, spastic pains in the various regions of the body and tissue systems.

b) Severe hunger as pathologic hunger.

c) Itching of certain areas of the body or certain spots of the body.

d) Disturbances in sleep occurring in the form of both difficulties in falling asleep and remaining asleep.

e) Fits of weakness.

f) Vomiting.

g) Fits of asthma.

h) Eruptions of sweat.

i) Fits of dizziness.

To a):

Pains occurring daily at a certain time somewhere in the body should prompt the doctor to check on the organ clock as to the respective organ and its maximum time. These pains may occur far remote from the actual location of the organ, which is in a state of incipient insufficiency.

Pains may occur:

1. Somewhere on the course of the meridian pertaining to the insufficient organ;

2. at the associated points of the organ meridian situated left and right to the vertebral column;

3. in a hyperalgetic zone pertaining to the insufficient organ according to *Head, Kappis-Laewen,* and *Lemaire;*

4. in circumscript muscular maximum points according to *Boas, Mussy-Westphal* and *Kohlrausch.*

Spastic pains in the abdomen occurring at certain times have different etiologies. The occurrence between 5 and 7 refers to spasms of the large intestine, and between 9 and 11 to spasms of the pancreas, and between 17 and 19 to spasms of the kidney, and between 23 and 1 to spasms of the gallbladder. When the doctor is called for a visit at one of these times, he should immediately be informed about the onset of such spastic pains, in order to obtain an etiologic hint as to the colic.

To b):

Severe hunger is a pathologic sign occurring not only in complaints of the stomach in incipient ulcer of the stomach. It mostly occurs in the maximum time of the stomach, but may also appear in the maximum time of a different organ (see case report No. 4 on page 134).

To c):

The occurrence of itching at particular spots of the body or circumscript areas of the body, at certain times, may serve as an etiologic hint. One should, further-more, find out about the directional course of the itching, in order to get a hint as to the meridian area, where the itching chiefly occurs. Thus, the occurring of itch-ing about 17.00 and somewhat later may, as often as not, refer to functional dis-turbances of the kidneys, and when the patient is asked about the location of the occurrence of this itching, one will almost exclusively get the answer that this itching is located at the inner side of the lower or upper leg, where the kidney meridian traverses.

To d):

Disturbances in sleep differ as to whether they are present in falling asleep or staying asleep. Both of these disturbances may be present simultaneously in patients, who are in very bad shape. One should make sure about the presence of difficulties in staying asleep, in order to obtain etiologic hints.

When a patient cannot fall asleep, one should be aware of the fact that coffeine or teaine not only affect the brain but also the endocrine glands whose maximum time is between 21.00 to 23.00.

When a patient goes to bed between 21.00 and 22.00 to wake up between 24.00 and 0.30, this is indicative of a biliary disturbance, since this is the maximum time of the gallbladder.

When the patient wakes up between 2.00 and 3.00 during the maximum time of the liver, a hepatic disturbance is to be expected.

Waking up about 3.30 indicates that a pulmonary insufficiency is present, and it should be noted that cardio-pulmonary insufficiency as an insufficiency of the right heart may lead to disturbances in sleep during that time.

To e):

Fits of weakness, that is, cardiac attacks not only occur during the maximum time of the heart between 11.00 to 13.00, but also at different times, such as be-fore and after midnight (see case report No. 7 on page 135). Circulatory weak-ness mostly occurs in the evening hours, that is, between 19.00 to 21.00.

To f):

Vomiting may occur at any time, by day and by night. In the morning it is due to the stomach, at noon it is due to the duodenum. Vomiting at night should always be associated with the exact time of its occurrence. For example: A patient came to see me whom I had treated previously for his duodenal ulcer stating that he had vomited at two o'clock at night. My first question was to find out what he had eaten in the evening and he reported that he had eaten a lobster cocktail in a pub. But already on the way home he nauseated and became giddy. Since the occurrence of the vomiting was in the maximum time of the liver between 1.00 and 3.00 at night, I associated this with an intoxication of the liver. The day before, he enjoyed perfect wellbeing and only after eating lobsters his complaints set in; this is what made me think of an infection of botulism. Thus, it turned out that the nosode of botulism D 3 was capable of balancing the measurement points of the liver, of the circulation, and of the heart. This showed, that my suspicion was correct.

To g):

Fits of asthma should be analyzed as to their actual time of occurrence. For example: A female patient of 26 years of age complained about fits of asthma occurring in the evening about 20.00, that is, the maximum time of circulation. There are no fits at night nor in the morning nor during daytime. The occurrence of fits of asthma during the maximum time of the circulation made me suspect a noxa affecting the circulation. On the measurement points for the gallbladder and the biliary pathways, and on the 3rd liver point as well as on the bronchi I found indicator drops, which could not only be removed by Coffea D 4, but the measurement values themselves of these organs went down to 50. When asked, the patient admitted that she drinks coffee each afternoon. The homeopathic preparation of Coffea was potentized up to D 200 and the patient was forbidden to drink coffee any longer, which achieved that the patient got rid of her fits of asthma. Today, this patient very occasionally drinks a cup of coffee, which does no longer affect her to cause fits of asthma.

To h):

Outbreaks of sweat may occur during different times at night. The beginning of sweating between 0.30 to 1.00 at night indicates that a biliary disturbance may be present. Sweating in the morning about 6.00 is always an indication that something is wrong with the large intestine or sections of it. Sweating in the early hours of the morning about 4.00 are mostly due to pulmonary disturbances.

130

To i):

Fits of dizziness. The time of occurrence of fits of dizziness may give important etiologic hints. The following case report may illustrate this:

A patient, 81 years of age, has consulted me for 20 years because of his chronic bronchitis and chronic pyelonephritis. Now, he complains about fits of dizziness after the intake of his breakfast. At 9 o'clock in the morning the patient's blood pressure is 160/90. There is no dizziness at night nor when he rises in the morning, nor when he changes the position of his body. No dizziness when looking upwards or downwards. The measurement points of the stomach are normal. Only the MP. Coeliac plexus shows an indicator drop on both sides of 86/76. To balance the values of the coeliac plexus down to 50, Terebinthina D 10 was required. So, I asked the question, if the patient inhaled any substance before having breakfast. He confirmed this and he brought his inhalant along with him. I found terpentine to be one component of the inhalant. By means of the saliva, part of the inhalant reached the stomach irritating in particular the coeliac plexus. From there, the labyrinth was irritated and caused dizziness after breakfast. After abandoning the inhalant, the patient has been free from fits of dizziness for three years now.

A number of case reports should give support to the above outlines:

Case report No. 1 – Intermittent fits of migraine.

A patient, 62 years of age, complains about the occurrence of migraine on the left side only. These fits have been present for more than 8 years occurring several times per week. Migraine appears at night during the time between 2.30 to 3.00 but, during the recent half year, the time of appearance has shifted to between 5.00 and 6.00. It was interesting to note, that according to the anamnesis of the patient, there have been no fits of migraine during the day-time. The occurrence about 2.30 is a hint to expect a hepatic insufficiency, the maximum time of the liver being between 1.00 and 3.00. The occurrence between 5.00 and 7.00 is an indication as to an insufficiency of the large intestine. The patient states however, that his stools are regular and painless.

Electro-acupuncture diagnostics reveal that both control measurement points (CMPs) of the liver show values of 80/64. Nosodes required for the 2nd liver measurement point were: Nosode of Hepatitis, nosode of Leptospirosis canicola, nosode of Leptospirosis icterohaemorrhagica, nosode of Listeriosis and Pasteurellosis, as well as nosode of Malaria, Malaria tropica, and of Yellow fever in addition of the nosode of Echinococcinum.

Furthermore, nine different potentized substances of the citric acid cycle were tested to be useful.

On the 3rd liver measurement point a number of insecticides were tested, these being:
KI 1, KI 2, KI 3, KI 4, KI 5, KI 14, KI 15, KI 16".

The control measurement point (CMP.) of the large intestine exhibited only an indicator drop of 89/70 on the left side. On the right side of the large intestine there was no indicator drop present. The four distal measurement points of the large intestine showed no indicator drops on the left side, but there was an indicator drop (ID.) of 88/70 on the measurement point for the peritoneum of the large intestine.

The following nosodes were required for balancing the measurement point of the peritoneum of the large intestine: Nosode of Peritonitis D 4, nosode of Shiga Kruse D 4, nosode of Dysenteria D 5.

Disturbances of the peritoneum of the small intestine could be balanced on the measurement point Peritoneum by the nosode of Peritonitis D 8, of Dysenteria D 10, of Shiga Kruse D 8. The patient had contracted dysentery twice during the war.

An inflammation of a peritoneal adhesion after approximate. 15 to 20 years of the actual acute disease, is sometimes the late after-effect of an overcome dysentery. I have seen this situation many times.

It was interesting, that during treatment the patient had migraine at 0.30 at night. This is the maximum time for the gallbladder. The reason for this was the palatable French cheese which the patient had eaten while on an official stay in France lasting several days. Thus, I was able to test the nosode of Lamblia intestinalis. Lamblia may often be found in French cheese which, in contrast to German cheese, need not be pasteurized to give a better taste.

Until December 19, 1974 the patient had received five injections of the mesenchyme reactivation cure. He came to see me on January 17, 1975 and reported that up to January 4, 1975 he had no more fits of migraine. At noon of this day, however, he had another first fit of migraine associated with fierce pains in the region of the heart. This I had never seen before for eight years. I started thinking of the reason for this in terms of chemical substances to irritate the heart during its maximum time in addition to disturbing the brain. This substance could only be cyanic acid. The preparation of Acidum hydrocyanicum D 4 tested on the measurement point Coronary vessels of the heart proved this. The patient who is fond of marzipan had eaten a lot of it when he was invited to friends of his the night before.

KI 1	Dichlorvos and Methoxychlor	KI 5	Hexacyclohexane comp. B
KI 2	Hexacyclohexane	KI 14	2 4 5 T-Ester
KI 3	Phosphor. acidester	KI 15	Paraquart
KI 4	Hexacyclohexane comp. A	KI 16	Toxa

Furthermore, the patient reported that on January 6. 9. 11. and 13. 1975. before 3.00 at night he had fits of migraine but no more as severely as before. This corresponded to the maximum time of the liver. The 1. MP. Allergy. left side. showed values of 80/60 and 89/70 on the right side. The other allergy points exhibited no indicator drops. This lead to the conclusion that the allergen could only have been taken by mouth. These two points were balanced by Urethanum D 3. The patient admitted that on the evenings preceding the fits of migraine he had drunk wine. which had apparently been added a chemical substance against turbidity.

To do this. had been legal in 1971 and 1972 and is no longer legal to-day. This chemical substance is broken down in the body to form urethane. which is carcinogenic affecting also the liver. which accounts for the fact that the light fits of migraine appeared at the maximum time of the liver. So. I advised the patient to refrain from drinking any wine while receiving the mesenchyme reactivation cure.

Case report No. 2 – Cramps in the abdomen.

A female patient. aged 26. gets cramps in the abdomen between 14.30 and 15.00 in the afternoon starting in the upper abdomen and pulling down to the urinary bladder. Furthermore. pains appear in the shoulder joint. left posterior side. also on the course of the small intestine meridian. The beginning of the abdominal cramps coincides with the maximum time of the small intestine. The patient was also suffering from a disturbance in the small intestine in the form of an inflammation of *Meckel's* diverticle. The following nosodes were tested:

Nosode of *Meckel's* Diverticle D 3 on the measurement point Ileum in addition to the nosode of Lymphangitis mesenterica D 3 on the measurement point for the Mesenterial lymph glands.

The pulling sensation of the pains from the upper abdomen to the urinary bladder was due to a long existing severely irritated urinary bladder. Already in May 1973. the patient had a papilloma of the urinary bladder removed. but the irritation in the urinary bladder remained to be present.

Case report No. 3 – Pains in the upper abdomen.

A female patient. aged 71. complains about abdominal pains occurring in the early morning hours between 5.00 and 6.00. that is the maximum time of the large intestine. particularly in the left upper abdomen.

Electro-acupuncture diagnostics reveal a motor insufficiency of the left colonic flexure. which was measured on the MP. Left colonic flexure   3   Large intestine point. left side. The left Colonic flexure in adults mostly exhibits an acute angle. In some cases. both sides of the flexure tend to lie even parallel (so-called twin-rifle shape).

Case report No. 4 – Severe hunger.

A girl, aged 15, gets a craving for sweets around 17.00 every day. Associated with this are fits of slight dizziness. In order to satisfy her hunger, she has to eat large amounts of sweets.

The maximum time of the kidney lies between 17.00 to 19.00. In acupuncture, the kidney is closely associated with the adrenal gland. For this reason I have checked the blood pressure on this girl. At 16.30 the blood pressure on the left side was at 120/70 and on the right side 135/75. This proved a unilateral disease of the right adrenal gland.

The MP. Adrenal gland = 10b. Kidney showed no indicator drop, however, the MP. Medulla of the adrenal gland = 10a. Kidney exhibited a value of 80/70. Typhinum D 6 balanced the points to 50. After carrying out a mesenchyme reactivation cure the severe hunger had gone and the blood pressure became normal on both sides at 110/80 taken in the afternoon at 17.00.

Case report No. 5 – Difficulties in falling asleep.

A 29 year old patient cannot fall asleep until 24.00 midnight in spite of having gone to bed at 22.00. Since these difficulties in falling asleep are in the maximum time of the triple-warmer, i.e., the endocrine system, I checked, first of all, the endocrine glands to find that the measurement values of the pituitary gland were 76/70 on the right side and 66/60 on the left side. The right pituitary gland required Tularemia D 6 to be balanced and the left pituitary gland required Toxoplasmosis D 4 to be balanced.

Tularemia is known for occassionally causing cerebral and encephalitic as well as meningitic symptoms (Sturm). In the postnatal form of acquired Toxoplasmosis a non-purulent encephalomyelitis or encephalitis of the medulla may occur. Since, however, the difficulties to fall asleep extend into the maximum time of the gallbladder function (biliary ducts and body of the gallbladder), I checked on the biliary ducts and the gallbladder measurement points to find a chronic cholangitis.

Functional biliary disturbances causing difficulties in falling asleep are very frequent. One should always bear in mind that the gallbladder meridian contains the measurement points for the function of the diencephalon and the mesencephalon. This is the reason why functional disturbances in the biliary system may likewise affect the sleep centers in the diencephalon and in the mesencephalon.

Case report No. 6 – Disturbances in sleep caused by the brain stem.

A 37 year old female patient suffering from allergy and migraine tended to fall a-sleep in the morning around 5.00 only. She used to lie in her bed wide awake as if she had drunk coffee. I was able to establish a disturbance of the gallbladder functions causing remote effects on the diencephalon's and mesenchephalon's sleep centers. Furthermore, I found considerable disturbances caused by toxins in the liver cell of toxoplasmosis, tularemia, listeriosis and pasteurellosis, which I could check on the 2nd Liver measurement point. In addition, in order to balance the 3rd Liver measurement point for the periportal tissue I found Penicillinum D 4 and Streptomycinum D 6.

On the allergy points of this patient I tested Acidum hydrocyanicum D 8 and Thio-urea D 4. The patient was fond of marzipan (cyanic acid) and oranges (preserva-tives). After balancing the two 3. Liver measurement points with the aid of Penicillinum D 4 and Streptomycinum D 6, the measurement values for the two sleep centers also went down to 50.

To balance the biliary functional dusturbances the following preparations were required:

Vegetable fat D 8, Coffea D 5, Magnesium muriaticum D 6 as well as the poten-tized substances of the intermediary fatty metabolism, that is, Acetone, Acetic Acid Ethylester, Glycerin, Cystinum, Cysteinum, all as D 8, in addition to Choles-terinum D 10.

This case constitutes the prototype of a severe disturbance in falling asleep with organ malfunctions lying in close succession as to the maximum times of the or-gan clock. These malfunctions being: Disturbances of the gallbladder, of the liver as well as a cardio-pulmonary insufficiency caused by a severe allergy which manifested itself in the maximum time between 3.00 and 5.00.

Case report No. 7 – Nocturnal cardiac attacks.

Female patient, aged 67, sufferring from hypertension suddenly experienced daily cardiac attacks occurring between 0.00 and 0.30. Since the cardiac attacks occur in the maximum time of the gallbladder, the biliary functions were ex-amined to show indicator drops on all points. In addition to the nosode of Cholangitis D 3 followed by the accompanying (complementary) medication of Colocynthis D 4, Chelidonium D 4, Carduus marianus D 4, Allium cepa D 4 could be verified. When asked, the patient confirmed that on the afternoon before the occurrence of the cardiac attacks she had eaten two large pieces of onion cake in addition to a Berliner (fried pancake). This was sufficient to boost up the latent biliary malfunction causing these nocturnal disturbances. This case report may give a typical proof for the midday-midnight rule, which implies that when an organ is in trouble, the organ following 12 hours later in the maximum time cycle will also be in danger.

Case report No. 8 – Disturbances in staying asleep.

A 54 year old patient complains about disturbances during sleep. After falling a-sleep at night he wakes up 1 and $1^1/_2$ hours later unable to fall asleep again and staying awake between 24.00 and 4.00 in the morning. This is the maximum time of the gallbladder and the liver. In search of biliary and hepatic disturbances I was able to find:

1. A chronic inflammation of the biliary pathways associated with disturbances in emptying the body of the gallbladder.
2. A severe allergy, in particular on the two 2nd Allergy measurement points, thus revealing that the allergy was based on inhalants.
3. A considerable insufficiency of the liver.

In my search for inhaled allergens I learnt, that in the house of the patient a flower-bed in one of his rooms had to be tightened by Inertol and Encalit. The whole house smelled of this material. The inhabitants of the house complained about burning eyes, disturbances in sight, and headaches. To account for the toxicity of the inhalent allergen I tested Anthracinum D 6, Pix crudum D 6 and KI 6 D 6 (Dinitrocresol). After that, not only were the allergy points balanced, but also the measurement values for the interior eye portions subsided from 86 to 66 on both sides.

Because of the severe allergy, the patient, for the support of his liver functions, was administered the eight substances of the potentized citric cycle in potencies of D 6, furthermore, because of the insufficiency of the biliary pathways he was administered the nosode of chronic Cholecystitis D 4, Enterococcinum D 4, Coli D 3, Proteus D 3, Aerobacter cum coli D 3, and Lamblia intestinalis D 3. As an accompanying (complementary) therapy Natrium choleinicum D 4, Mercurius dulcis D 5, Ornithogalum D 5, Benzochinon D 5, Viscum Betulae D 5 were applied. After this, the disturbances of sleep had disappeared after a short while.

Case report No. 9 – Permanent pains flaring up between 19.00 and 21.00 hours.

This case report, again, shows that in multiple complaints of a 62 year old female patient lasting for the whole day each day with varying intensity it may be useful to find out about the time of the maximum occurrence of complaints. The patient

136

suffered from headaches, dizziness, oppression around the heart, post-sternal pains and disturbances in sight in the form of lateral deviation of the straight-on sight (forward vision), as well as cramps in the stomach and in the oesophagus. Although these complaints lasted more or less for the whole day, the worst occurrance was between 19.00 and 21.00, that is, the maximum time of the circulation. This gave me a hint as to what I had to search for in this patient. The measurement values on the summation measurement point (SMP.) Arteries were 92/76 on both sides.

Both measurement points for the internal ear exhibited values of 100. For the circulation, I tested the nosode of Botulism D 3, for the internal ear the nosode of Botulism D 6, and for the measurement point RES. = (reticulo-endothelial system) the nosode of Botulism D 12 together with the corresponding accompanying (complementary) therapy, i.e., Aranea diadema D 4, Triticum repens D 3, Calcium picrinicum D 6, Calcium phosphoricum D 6. The patient rapidly got rid of her complaints. Since in this case the most severe complaints were between 19.00 and 21.00, that is, the maximum time of the circulation, I was led on my way to search for botulism, which may have a considerable impact on the circulatory centers situated in the brain stem.

Differential diagnosis as to the presence of ventricular ulcer and duodenal ulcer based on the temporal occurrence of complaints in the maximum times.

The differential diagnosis of ulcers in the stomach and in the duodenum should always refer to the maximum times of the stomach and small intestine. Complaints about a stomach ulcer are predominantly in the morning between 7.00 and 9.00. Complaints about the duodenal ulcer are in the afternoon between 13.00 and 15.00. When, during the maximum time of the small intestine, complaints in the upper abdomen are localized on the left side, irritational states of the ascending part of the duodenum associated with corresponding functional disturbances should be considered. The ascending part of the duodenum, in particular, is responsible for the secretion of serotonin. This is why patients suffering from the sudden release of serotonin between 13.00 and 15.00 complain about severe pains in the upper abdomen associated with a rise in blood pressure as well as headaches.

The use of the maximum time for a specific application of medications.

When the disturbance of an organ does not affect the entire function yet, that is, when a pre-insufficiency or an incipient insufficiency is present, this organ will first of all manifest symptoms in the maximum time. For the medical doctor this is an indication, in order to cope with these complaints, to apply a corresponding medication one to two hours prior to the maximum time in favour of the damaged organ. This will achieve, that when the maximum time of the organ occurs, the organ has received some support already. The application of medications on the basis of the maximum times and the minimum times of organs will frequently require an additional administration of medications on top of the usual medications to be taken three times a day before or after meals.

Thus, the patient suffering from disturbances in sleep between 12 a.m. to 1 a.m. should get a specific remedy for the gallbladder function before going to bed, that is, about 10 to 10.30 p.m. The patient suffering from an insufficiency of the right heart should have a remedy available next to his bed to be taken at 3.00 after waking up in order to abridge the period of weakness by this additional therapy. The additional administration of medications during the day time according to the maximum times of the organs can be carried out without difficulties as long as the patient will take the medication at the prescribed time. It is interesting to note that orthodox clinical experiences in the optimal administration of specific remedies with respect to the maximum time of the pancreas are available. A diabetic should take his antidiabetic remedies or inject the insulin in the morning between 7.00 and 9.00, that is before the maximum time of the pancreas. When considering the maximum times of organs, one will only observe the daily regular occurrence of complaints in disturbed organ functions without being able to associate these complaints with an organ itself. This however, must be taken as an early symptom for preventive measures.

Electro-acupuncture diagnostics may verify these hints immediately in the early phases of deficiencies.

Finally, the following outlines should be made on the maximum times:

1. For the Chinese organ clock or the maximum times the respective local time should be applied, i.e., the medium solar time applicable to all places of the same degree of longitude. Regional time, in contrast, refers to larger areas depending on the average local time. For example, in Germany, Central European Time is used corresponding to 15 degrees of Eastern longitude passing through Greenwich.

2. The maximum time lasting for two hours has a peak of energy flow in the middle, that is one hour after the beginning of the maximum time on the even hour. This is supported by the observation that in an incipient insufficiency complaints occur only after the expiration of one hour of the maximum time. When the organ insufficiency has progressed to a major degree complaints will occur sooner, that is, after half an hour or immediately at the beginning of the maximum time.

3. In addition to the maximum time of the organs, there is the minimum time of the organs shifted by twelve hours on the organ clock (in juxta-position). The minimum time may become important when the insufficiency of an organ in the maximum time coincides with an insufficiency of an organ in the minimum time.

138

Coincidence of two functional organ disturbances in the maximum- and the minimum time.

Please refer to case report No. 7 concerning nocturnal cardiac attacks. This is a typical example for the coincidence of two organ insufficiencies both in the maximum – and in the minimum time. An organ insufficiency does not assure the sufficient production of energy for an organ in its maximum time, that is, the organ will experience an energetic deficiency. This will manifest itself either by disturbances in the organ itself or on the course of the organ meridian including the areas left and right to that meridian.

Simultaneously, the organ which has been affected, will also make itself felt in its minimum time, since the reduced formation of energy likewise is not sufficient for the energetic supply to the organ in its minimum time.

Maximum time	Minimum time
Heart	Gallbladder
Small intestine	Liver
Urinary bladder	Lung
Kidney	Large intestine
Circulation	Stomach
Triple-warmer	Spleen-pancreas
Gallbladder	Heart
Liver	Small intestine
Lung	Urinary bladder
Large intestine	Kidney
Stomach	Circulation
Spleen-pancreas	Triple-warmer

Case report No. 7 shows that acute biliary functional disturbances around midnight may simultaneously trigger a cardiac attack in a chronically damaged heart. After the intake of a large quantity of fatty food in the evening an insufficient heart in its minimum time may suffer a cardiac infarction at the maximum time of the gallbladder.

Just to add same further examples:

In a functional disturbance of the small intestine associated with insufficient fermentation with a hepatic functional disturbance being present at the same time, the patient will exhibit at night between 1 to 3 a.m., that is during the maximum time of the liver, disturbances in sleep in addition to strong meteoristic complaints.

When a cardio-pulmonary insufficiency interrupts the sleep at night between 3 to 5 a.m. and when there is simultaneously an insufficiency of the urinary bladder or a genito-urinary functional disturbance, the patient will feel at the same time severe vesical irritations.

When a patient suffering from a diverticulitis in the large intestine wakes up between 5.00 and 7.00 in the morning with a renal functional disturbance being present simultaneously, pains in the kidneys will occur during this time as well. A patient suffering from a gastric ulcer in addition to disturbances of circulation, will complain about his stomach in the morning in addition to bodily weakness and dizziness, occurring at the same time.

Intestinal disturbances after the midday meal indicate an insufficiency of the small intestine during its maximum time between 1 to 3 p.m. Tiredness after the midday meal with insufficiency of the liver leading to acute tiredness after the intake of food, is based on the minimum time of the insufficient liver.

Insufficiency of the pancreas in its maximum time between 9 to 11 a.m. with endocrine insufficiency existing simultaneously will lead to a lack of energy and drive, i.e., during the minimum time of the endocrine gland.

Are there any exceptions to the rule of the maximum time?

A vagotonic person makes an exception. His rhythm of life is somewhat changed. In the morning he needs a much longer starting time and does not get active before ten in the morning. But he is surprisingly active in the evening, when other people become tired and go to bed. Such vagotonic persons tend to go to bed at midnight or later. Considering the rule of the maximum times concerning vagotonic people, one will find that the maximum times have shifted by one or two hours, in other words, the maximum time occurs later. In that case, the maximum time for the large intestine is between 7 to 9 a.m. when stools will be discharged. The maximum time of the stomach is between 9 to 11 a.m. and this is when a vagotonic person feels hungry. When these people have to take breakfast earlier in the morning they only tend to drink a little without eating anything. When they have a chance, these people will postpone their midday meal until the early afternoon. The maximum time of the triple-warmer is between 11 p.m. and 1 a.m. This is why the vagotonic person goes to bed after midnight while the normal person, after his maximum time of the triple-warmer, goes to bed at 10 p.m.

Effects of the maximum times on man working at night.

Since in persons working during day time an incipient insufficiency of the gallbladder, the liver, and the lung leads to disturbances in sleep of various kinds, these disturbances have to be remembered as occurring only during the phase of rest.

140

For men working at night these disturbances should occur much more severely. From experience we know that men working at night should only eat very limited portions of meal. Furthermore, it is an empiric fact that somebody working regularly at night is much better off healthwise than someone working intermittently early, or late- and on night shift.

Additional final remark.

Maximum times may serve as diagnostic hints for the etiology of unresolved complaints as well as an early diagnosis for incipient insufficiencies of an organ facilitating preventive therapy of pre-insufficiencies by the consulting doctor.

Minimum times of organs in minimal organ functions have to be considered in addition to the presence of further functional organ disturbances as diagnostic hints in pluri-morbid patients.

Maximum and minimum times of an organ may be compared with the oceanic tides. High tides or flood up to the highest mark corresponding to the energic maximum in the middle of the two-hour maximum time; low waters or ebb to the lowest mark corresponding to the energetic minimum in the middle of the two-hour minimum time.

Rules of the energy exchange.

The rules of the energy exchange in classical acupuncture can only be applied after carrying out pulse diagnoses in order to prick the correct acupuncture points. The following rules apply:

1. Rule of mother and son
2. Rule of husband and housewife
3. Rule of the coupled meridians (corresponding organs)
4. Rule of midnight – midday.

1. Rule of mother and son.

The rule of mother and son should be applied when a weak organ cannot be tonified by means of the customary points. The preceding organ in the energy cycle which is denoted as mother has to be tonified, while the organ following the weak organ is denoted as son and should be sedated. The rule of mother and son is based on the succession of the organs in the energy cycle according to the maximum times.

When applying the rule of mother and son in a treatment of the heart, the spleen-pancreas meridian and the small intestine meridian have to be treated, both of which have an important function in the formation of ferments for breaking down nutritional agents and for changing the energy. A sufficient energy production is one of the pre-requisites for an optimal heart function. In practice, one may treat both spleen-pancreas and small intestine to apply therapy to the heart. A successful treatment of this kind may always be verified by electro-acupuncture as to the heart.

In a functional disturbance of the kidneys one will treat, according to the rule of mother and son, the urinary bladder as a preceding organ and the circulation as a successive organ. In acupuncture, the meridian of the urinary bladder with its 67 points is of greatest importance. The urinary bladder not only constitutes a hollow organ to assemble the urine from the kidneys but also cares for the energetic supply and the steering of the entire genito-urinary area. A strengthening of the urinary bladder's function and of the entire genito-urinary organs results in an accelerated lymphatic drainage of the minor pelvis, which in turn improves the lymphatic supply of the kidneys. The treatment of the circulation promotes the arterial vasculation and removes spasms of the renal arteriols in kidney diseases which results in a better concentration function of the kidney. These two examples may suffice to make clear that the application of the rule of mother and son coincides with effects of clinical experiences.

The rule of mother and son as a functional energetic succession according to the energetic flooding of the organs, enables the medical doctor to treat the additional organs preceding or following in the energy cycle when a damaged organ does not respond to therapy.

2. The rule of husband and housewife as a law for the parallel relations between the left and the right pulses.

The rule of husband and housewife is based on the energetic relations of organs of adjacent anatomic pulses. The three pulses situated on the left and right radial artery respectively are diagnosed according to their superficial or deeper positions, each organ corresponding to one position. The anatomic positions of the three pulse loci:

I. Pulse locus between apophysis and wrist joint, that is, distally to the apophysis.

II. Pulse locus situated on the apophysis itself.

III. Pulse locus proximally to the apophysis.

On the left side superficial and deep pulses are distinguished. On the right side as to the second and third pulse locus one differs between a superficial, a middle, and a deep pulse.

Position of the organs as to the left pulses:

I. Superficial: Small intestine – deep: Heart

II. Superficial: Gallbladder – deep: Liver

III. Superficial: Urinary bladder – deep: Kidney.

Positions of the organs as to the right pulses:

I. Superficial: Large intestine – deep: Lung

II. Superficial: Stomach – middle: Pancreas – deep: Spleen

III. Superficial: Triple-warmer – middle: Circulation – deep: Sexual organs.

Thus, the Yang organs possess superficial pulses and the Yin organs one deep, and one middle, and one deep pulse. The rule of the husband and housewife implies that when an organ, whose pulse is situated on the left hand, gets sick, the organ situated on the corresponding pulse locus on the right hand gets into danger (see the dotted lines on page 103). The following table may illustrate this:

Sick organ:	In danger:
Small intestine	Large intestine
Heart	Lung
Gallbladder	Stomach
Liver	Pancreas or spleen
Urinary bladder	Triple-warmer (endocrine organs)
Kidney	Circulation and sexual organs.

The rule of husband and housewife is a preventive law in acupuncture indicating the organ in danger because of another sick organ. This is important for the medical doctor to carry out preventive medicine. This rule, furthermore, documents the superiority of the male principle (organs on the left side) over the female principle (organs on the right pulse loci) in acupuncture.

Thousands of electro-acupuncture measurements, however, showed, that the superiority of the organs on the left side with respect to the rule husband – housewife in classical acupuncture is not true. Since one may equally reverse this rule in that a sick organ on the right pulse locus may involve corresponding organs of the pulse locus on the left hand. So, diseases of organs situated on the right side necessitate the preventive treatment of the corresponding organ on the left side as well. The following organs should be treated when one organ is sick:

Sick organ:	To be treated as well:
Large intestine	Small intestine
Lung	Heart
Stomach	Gallbladder
Spleen-pancreas	Liver
Triple-warmer	Urinary bladder
Circulation	Kidney.

Also from a clinical point of view these relations, as stated above, can be explained: When the large intestine gets sick, the small intestine will follow since dysbacteria of the large intestine travels upwards to the small intestine. In pulmonary diseases the right heart in particular will be affected.

Disturbances of the stomach will also involve the functions of the gallbladder which in particular is the case in subacidity or anacidity of the stomach. The infectious germs travel from the stomach to the duodenum and to the biliary pathways to maintain a chronic cholangitis.

A disease of the pancreas associated with insufficient fermentation and repercussions on the intermediary metabolism of protein, carbohydrate, fats, and uric acid, because of insufficient breakdown of the substances, will likewise involve the liver which in turn has to cope with a larger quantity of semifinished products of the intermediary metabolism. Endocrine insufficiencies affect the genito-urinary organs, in particular the prostate, which belongs to the urinary bladder in acupuncture. Vascular diseases associated with mural changes and spasms affect the renal arteriols thus impeding the concentration function of the kidneys.

Summary:

In observing the rule of husband – housewife in its enlarged form, as stated above, the medical doctor in addition to treating the sick organ may simultaneously apply preventive therapy on the corresponding organ in danger.

The rule of crosswise relations between the left and the right pulse loci.

There exist the following relations between the superficial pulse loci (see Figure on page 103 in particular the lines between the organs).

a) Small intestine (first pulse locus on the left side) related to the triple-warmer or endocrine meridian (third pulse locus on the right side).

b) Gallbladder (second pulse locus on the left side) related to the large intestine (first pulse locus on the right side).

c) Urinary bladder (third pulse locus on the left side) related to the stomach (second pulse locus on the right side).

The following pathologic explanations may back these relations:

to a):

In insufficient ferment production of the small intestine the transformation of food stuffs into energy is insufficient as well. Therefore, the endocrine system does not receive an adequate amount of energy, which results in functional insufficiency.

to b):

An insufficient secretion of the gall into the duodenum causes a lack of cholic acids to stimulate the motility of the large intestine.

to c):

In an insufficient function of the urinary bladder the stomach will become suboranacid, or even suffer from subfermentation or nonfermentation.

There exist the following relations originating from the deep pulse loci:

a) Heart (first pulse locus left side) to the circulation (third pulse locus on the right side).

b) Liver (second pulse locus on the left side) to the lung (first pulse locus on the right side).

c) Kidney (third pulse locus on the left side) to the spleen-pancreas (second pulse locus on the right side).

For this, the following pathologic explanations may be given:

to a):

Disturbances of the heart lasting for a long period of time involve the circulatory system.

to b):

In insufficient detoxification of the liver part of the toxins is excreted via the mucous membranes of the respiratory passages. This is why in chronic refractory bronchitis intensive therapy of the liver should be carried out.

to c):

Insufficient renal function, among other things, results in insufficient secretion of uric acid. Uric acid remains in the body depositing there. Because of the increased amount of uric acid in the body, the formation of the ferment of nuclease in the pancreas is lagging behind.

As a sign of insufficiency of the spleen, lymphatic oedemas may arise such as in the face below the eyes.

Repetitive remarks: As to the patho-physiologic significance of the crossed relations between pulse loci, one has to concede that the pulse loci on the left side exercise a major influence. There do exist exceptions however, when the pulse loci on the right side are predominant.

3. Rule of the coupled organs (corresponding organs)

This is a law of interrelations in acupuncture for

1. preventive treatment and
2. treatment of a coupled organ when organ therapy otherwise does not respond.

I have outlined on this already in the Textual Volume I on the Topographic Positions of the Measurement Points in Electro-Acupuncture on page 104. When the Yang organ of an organ pair is sick, its coupled Yin organ is in danger and vice versa. This is the situation of the endangered corresponding organ. In classical acupuncture as a preventive measure, the passage points of these organs have to be needled.

The below Yin organs have the following corresponding organs:

Heart	the Yang organ of the small intestine
Kidney	the Yang organ of the urinary bladder
Liver	the Yang organ of the gallbladder
Lung	the Yang organ of the large intestine
Spleen-pancreas	the Yang organ of the stomach.

The circulation as a functional steering system has the triple-warmer = endocrine system as a corresponding organ and as a functional steering system alike.

Also, in medication therapy the heart may be treated successfully via the small intestine. The improvement of fermentation resulting in an increase of energy formation has a favourable effect on the function of the heart.

In diseases of the kidney the treatment of the urinary bladder and the genito-urinary organs will be favourable for functions of the kidneys.

When the liver is sick, the restitution of an optimal function of the biliary system will be of great advantage.

To improve the dysbacteria of the intestine is favourable for the functions of the lung. In the thirties, when tuberculostatic medications were missing, tuberculosis of the lungs was taken care of in the various sanatoria by treating the dysbacteria of the intestine.

The below Yang organs have the following corresponding organs:

Small intestine	the Yin organ of the heart
Urinary bladder	the Yin organ of the kidney
Gallbladder	the Yin organ of the liver
Large intestine	the Yin organ of the lung
stomach	the Yin organs spleen and pancreas considered in acupuncture as one single organ.

In diseases of the small intestine associated with special aggravation of functional disturbances during the maximum time, i.e., after lunch, and resulting in audible movements of the bowel even when lying down, an improvement of the output of the heart effecting a better vascularization of the intestinal organs will have a favourable effect on digestive processes.

In all inflammatory diseases of the urinary bladder the treatment of the renal pelvis which is mostly involved simultaneously, will be advantageous for the urinary bladder as well.

In inflammations of the biliary pathways associated with a swelling of the mucous membranes and thus a narrowing of the lumen of the draining biliary pathways as well as a retarded excretion of the bile into the duodenum, an improvement of the hepatic functions will promote the formation of the bile in the liver cells and, at the same time, increase the pressure of the secreted biliary liquids (vis-a-tergo).

In diseases of the large intestine the diaphragm will be pressed upwards due to the meteorism mostly existing simultaneously thus diminishing the vital capacity of the lungs.

In diseases of the stomach the improvement of the pancreatic functions, because of an augmented fermentation, will improve the digestive process, which otherwise is incomplete in the stomach.

Rule: Midnight – midday

According to this rule two organs are associated with each other differing only by twelve hours as to the Chinese organ clock (maximum times): A Yang-organ is opposed to a Yin-organ and vice versa; the time between midnight and midday is called Yang-time, while the time between midday and midnight is called Yin-time. This rule enables the needle acupuncturist to tonify a Yang-organ during the Yang-time and thereby sedate the corresponding Yin-organ. Thus, a tonification of the large intestine in the morning (Yang-time) will sedate the kidney as the organ in juxta-position. A stimulation of the large intestine promotes defecation to avoid solidification of the stools, which in turn sedates the renal function because of reduced liquid secretion.

A sedation of the Yin-organ in the afternoon (Yin-time) will tonify the corresponding Yang-organ in juxta-position. When sedating the kidneys in the afternoon, the large intestine will be tonified. Augmented renal secretion facilitates solidification of the liquid stools in the large intestine.

Comparison of organs according to the midnight-midday rule.

Yin-time	Opposition
1– 3 p.m. Small intestine	1– 3 a.m. Liver
3– 5 p.m. Urinary bladder	3– 5 a.m. Lung
5– 7 p.m. Kidney	5– 7 a.m. Large intestine
7– 9 p.m. Circulation	7– 9 a.m. Stomach
9–11 p.m. Triple-warmer	9–11 a.m. Spleen-pancreas
Transition of Yin- to Yang-time	
11 p.m.–1 a.m. Gallbladder	1 a.m.–1 p.m. Heart

Yang-time	
1– 3 a.m. Liver	1– 3 p.m. Small intestine
3– 5 a.m. Lung	3– 5 p.m. Urinary bladder
5– 7 a.m. Large intestine	5– 7 p.m. Kidney
7– 9 a.m. Stomach	7– 9 p.m. Circulation
9–11 a.m. Spleen-Pancreas	9–11 p.m. Triple-warmer
Transition of Yang- to Yin-time	
11 a.m.–1 p.m. Heart	11 p.m.–1 a.m. Gallbladder

How may this mutual influence be explained from a pathophysiologic point of view considering, for example, heart and gallbladder functions? By stimulating the heart, the liver's vascularization is improved thus promoting the biliary secretion of the hepatic cells into the biliary capillaries and draining the liver itself; this in turn will lower the diaphragm thus improving the function of the heart (chiefly on mechanistic observations). On the other hand, insufficient cardiac action will promote hepatic blocks, which will lift the diaphragm resulting again in decreased biliary secretion, worse intestinal action, and meteorism.

In diseases of the small intestine when associated with reduced ferment production the breaking down of the nutritional agents will remain incomplete resulting in an increase of intermediary metabolic products, which have to be detoxified by the liver.

In diseases of the urinary bladder associated with insufficient urine excretion, a retrograde stasis in the kidneys will result affecting the entire body. This may cause pulmonary stasis in the form of a more or less pronounced oedema of the lungs with blood plasma passing trans-cellularly into the alveols. A stimulation of the vesical functions will also drain the organs in the body.

In diseases of the kidney with reduced urine secretion, liquids will assemble in the large intestine. In stimulating the large intestine by medications to get rid of liquefied stools, one will take care of the kidneys as well.

Circulatory disturbances in hypotensive persons are usually associated with sub- or anacidity in the stomach. By treating hypotension, one will improve the action of the stomach.

Insufficient endocrine activity, among other things, promotes lymphatic blocks and reduces the immune response of the spleen. The following examples are given with respect to insufficient activity of the endocrine glands resulting in lymphatic blocks.

1. Myxoedema in thyroid insufficiency;
2. Tetany associated with oedemas in the hand, the feet, and the face in parathyroid insufficiency;
3. Pituitary insufficiency in girls and in climacteric women associated with oedemas in the lower legs and amenorrhoea.

When looking at the organs of the midnight-midday-rule, one will obtain the same result as in the juxta-positions of the maximum- and minimum times as on page 139.

When observing the midnight-midday-rule, one may often get diagnostic hints. For example: A 53 year old female patient complained about pains in the right groin in the evenings only, that is, between 21.00 and 23.00 after lying down. This accounts for endocrine weakness associated with tiredness and spleen-pancreas insufficiency. The minimum time of the spleen-pancreas in the above evening hours creates, as an early symptom of spleen-pancreas insufficiency, pain in the right groin, where EAV has its 2. MP. for the hip joint, this being the 11a. Spleen-pancreas point found by EAV. A specific therapy of the pancreas administered in the evening caused the pains in the groin to disappear rapidly.

Final remarks.

The various rules of the energy exchange in acupuncture may be taken advantage of by the medical doctor in his consulting hours in many respects:

1. As diagnostic hints and early diagnosis when complaints are present in the maximum time of organs facilitating early therapy by administering medications at certain times one to two hours before the maximum time.
2. The utilization of the rule of mother-and-son when a damaged organ does not respond to treatment.
3. For preventive treatment of an endangered organ using the rule of husband-and-housewife, enlarged also by the use of the rule starting on the right side and turning to the left side, furthermore, using the rule of crosswise relations between the left and right pulse loci.
4. The rule of midnight-midday points to the endangered organ in the minimum time, when an organ is diseased in its maximum time; this should lead to preventive therapy when this very organ has been pre-damaged.
5. For preventive therapy, furthermore, the endangered corresponding organ of an organ pair may be used.

Summary of the endangered organs for preventive therapy:
This summary is given by the following rules:
1. Rule of the coupled organs
2. Rule of husband-housewife in its enlarged form
3. Rule of midnight-midday
4. Rule of crosswise relations of the pulse loci.

In diseases of the heart	endangered organs: 1. Small intestine 2. Lungs 3. Gallbladder 4. Circulation
in diseases of the small intestine or duodenum	1. Heart 2. Large intestine 3. Liver 4. Endocrine system
in diseases of the urinary bladder or genito-urinary organs	1. Kidney 2. Triple-warmer 3. Spleen-pancreas 4. Stomach
in diseases of the kidney	1. Urinary bladder 2. Circulation sexual sphere 3. Large intestine 4. Spleen-pancreas
in diseases of the circulation	1. Triple-warmer 2. Kidneys 3. Stomach 4. Small intestine
in diseases of the triple-warmer or the endocrine glands	1. Circulation 2. Urinary bladder 3. Spleen-pancreas 4. Small intestine
in diseases of the gall-bladder or biliary pathways	1. Liver 2. Stomach 3. Heart 4. Large intestine

in diseases of the liver	1. Gallbladder
	2. Spleen-pancreas
	3. Small intestine
	4. Lungs

in diseases of the lungs	1. Large intestine
	2. Heart
	3. Urinary bladder
	4. Liver

in diseases of the large intestine	1. Lungs
	2. Small intestine
	3. Kidneys
	4. Gallbladder

in diseases of the stomach	1. Spleen-pancreas
	2. Gallbladder
	3. Circulation
	4. Urinary bladder

in diseases of the spleen-pancreas	1. Stomach
	2. Liver
	3. Triple-warmer
	4. Kidney

This summary shows that when one organ is diseased, four further organs are in danger, according to the teachings of acupuncture. By exclusively treating the four endangered organs the disease of the primary organ will benefit. It is obvious in acupuncture that there exist clear notions as to the mutual influence of diseases of organs. These criteria had to be established for the Chinese physician whose emphasis in medical action was on preventive medicine in that he was not payed for treating diseases but for maintaining health. When his preventive medical action was bad he had to treat for nothing. The doctor who had carried out the best preventive medicine had the least amount of work to do for treating diseases. These above acupuncture rules may be applied by any physician for preventive medicine in his daily office, even if he does not use acupuncture or electro-acupuncture. The maximum times may be used as diagnostic hints when complaints occur at regular certain times. The electro-acupuncturist may objectify the relations to the endangered organs by using certain measurement points of the damaged organ. In addition, he may control the success of his preventive medicine with respect to the damaged organ.

Results of therapy carried out exclusively on the four endangered organs in a functionally insufficient heart

In order to prove the therapeutic success in a functionally disturbed heart by treating the four endangered organs exclusively: small intestine, lung, gallbladder, and circulation, I carried out the following examinations prior to and after electro-acupuncture therapy on the measurement points by means of low frequency current impulses:

Measurement points	Measurement values	
Heart right side	prior to	after EAV-therapy
pulmonary valve	80	60
pericardium	82	62
tricuspid valve	82	64
conduction system	84	62
cardiac muscle	80/76	64
Heart left side		
aortic valve	80	60
pericardium	80	60
mitral valve	80	60
conduction system	80	60
cardiac muscle (myocardium)	80	60

Measurement values of the endangered organs prior to treatment

Small intestine and duodenum, right side

upper horizontal part of the duodenum	80
descending part of the duodenum	82
lower horizontal part of the duodenum	80
peritoneum of the duodenum	78
ileum, right side	78

Duodenum and small intestine, left side

ascending part of the duodenum	80
duodeno-jejunal flexure	80
peritoneum	82
ileum, left side	82

Lung	right	left
parenchyma of the lung	70	80
bronchioli	74	80
pleura	80	80
bronchi	84	80
trachea	80	80

Biliary pathways – body of the gallbladder, right side

choledochal duct	80
peritoneum of the gallbladder	80
cystic duct	82
body of the gallbladder	80
biliferous ductuli	80

Biliary pathways, left side

common hepatic duct	80
right hepatic duct	60
left hepatic duct	80
biliferous ductuli	80

Circulation	right	left
SMP. arteries	68	78
SMP. veins	84	82
coronary arteries	82	84

(SMP. = Summation measurement point)

By administering low frequency direct current impulses and using least current intensity on all measurement points of the endangered organs as indicated, i.e., small intestine, duodenum, lung, gallbladder, biliary pathways, and circulation, in order to balance all values down to 50, the measurement results of the measurement readings of the heart improved; the indicator drop on one measurement point of the heart disappeared, all of the measurement points of the right heart came down to values of 60; measurement values of the left heart had come down to 60 or 62. It was possible to harmonize the values between the left and the right side. The new measurement values could be achieved under EAV-therapy as shown above. It should be emphazised once more that the very measurement points of the heart itself were not treated. Only by treating the four endangered organs, the situation of the heart improved considerably.

Influence of the organ pairs on the tonsils, jaw sections, ear and paranasal sinus.

Each organ pair, furthermore, has an energetic influence on:

a) one of the paranasal sinuses or the ear;

b) one of the five tonsils of the lymphatic tonsillar ring;

c) one of the five jaw sections both in the upper and lower jaw.

To a)

Small intestine – heart influence the ear (see "Interrelations of odontons and tonsils to organs, fields of disturbance and tissue systems", ML Verlag, 1978, page 98).

Lung – large intestine influence the ethomoid cells (see page 169).

Gallbladder – liver influence the sphenoidal sinus (see page 171).

To b)

Small intestine – heart influence the lingual tonsil (see page 106).

Lung – large intestine influence the tubal tonsil (see page 102).

Gallbladder – liver influence the palatine tonsil (see page 98).

To c)

Small intestine – heart influence the 8th odonton in the upper and lower jaw (see page 34).

lung – large intestine influence the 6th and 7th odontons in the lower jaw and the 4th and 5th odontons in the upper jaw (see page 27).

gallbladder – liver influence the 3rd odonton in the upper and lower jaw (see page 25).

Further outlines on this are given in the book "Interrelations of Odontons and Tonsils to Organs, Fields of Disturbance, and Tissue Systems".

EAV-therapy of the four endangered organs in a functionally disturbed heart also resulted in an improvement of the values of the following cranial organs:

Measurement points	prior to the treatment		after EAV-therapy	
	right	left	right	left
middle ear	90	84	70	70
internal ear	90	84	70	70
ethmoid cells	90	86	70	70
sphenoidal cells	84	84	70	70
lingual tonsil	82	86/80	72	72
palatine tonsil	82	82/76	72	72

Jaw measurement values.

Prior to the treatment			following the treatment		
84	86	82	66	60	64
84	84	84	62	62	60

Short specific medication test

The busy doctor in his daily practice may carry out a short medication test and thus apply to the patient a strong impulse for improving to treat the diseased organ to be treated in addition to the four endangered organs. This short medication test is sufficient as a treatment for all slight and less severe cases provided that the pathologic disturbances are not being maintained by foci or fields of disturbance.

On the occasion of an introductory course in 1978 I demonstrated on a colleague in his fifties who was taking three capsules of Septacord daily for his heart that: Fagopyrum D 4 for the small intestine, Badiaga D 4 for the lung, Ptelea trifoliata D 3 for the gallbladder, Aranea diadema D 4 for the circulation caused all measurement points of the heart to get down to 50.

How is such an effect on the heart possible? By normalizing the three organs and the circulation, the resistances in these organs and in the circulation are being decreased and cancelled thus enabling the heart to fulfill its functions by using less strength without medications.

Conclusions

When the diseased organ is treated in addition to the four endangered organs, five main organs of the body will be normalized energetically thus resulting in a restitution of optimal organic functions.

This normalization will not be confined energetically to the main organs only but will also involve energetically the paranasal sinuses, the ear, the tonsils, and the jaw sections in that the measurement values of these organs will normalize as well.

Maximum times of organs in the annual rhythm (monthly maximum times).

Finally I should like to point out that monthly maximum times of organs may be derived from a number of observations applicable to man in the Northern hemisphere. These maximum times of organs are the following:

January	– Gallbladder
February	– Urinary bladder
March	– Stomach
April	– Large intestine
May	– Small intestine
June	– Triple-warmer
July	– Kidney
August	– Spleen
September	– Liver
October	– Circulation

| November | – Lungs |
| December | – Heart |

It is interesting to note in this summary that from January to July, that is, in the first half of the year, only Yang organs are mentioned, i.e., carvernous organs. In the second half of the year we find only Yin-organs, that is, parenchymal organs. I could imagine that the observation of the maximum times of organs in the various months may give occasional hints for the etiology of unresolved complaints of an incipient organic disease. Furthermore, in a predamaged patient one may carry out preventive therapy by applying at least four weeks before the maximum monthly time of the organ a certain therapy to fortify the organic function thus assuring that the maximum monthly time of the organ itself will pass without any major disturbances for the patient.

Part III

Choice of the Examination Place in Electro-acupuncture acc. to Voll (EAV)

Reasons for mistakes of the beginner in EAV.

Every new method is difficult in the beginning. This applies equally to EAV. EAV was introduced to the medical public for the first time on a seminar for empirical treatments in Limburg/Germany in March 1955. After the demonstration of the diagnostic means in EAV, more and more medical doctors came to acquaint themselves with the theoretic and practical background of this method. Many of those, who luckily were in the possession of an instrument, got disappointed, though, because of failures in electro-acupuncture diagnostics and therapy, i.e., treatment of pathologic values by means of low frequency impulses. When these colleagues followed my request to see me in Plochingen and to bring their instrument with them, I had to realize that the instruments worked properly.

First of all, I had to find out if the colleague was able to establish a faultfree diagnosis and to decrease elevated values by means of electro-acupuncture therapy. When reasons for mistakes could be excluded, the unsatisfactory function of the instrument in practical performance in the hands of the colleague could only be due to a localized disturbance to exclude the proper application of EAV. This turned out to be true in a few cases.

First of all, I had to advise on carrying out test measurements in a different room of the medical office or in the private rooms of the medical doctor. Then, in several cases, EAV could be carried out.

It also happened that an examination in the office could not be done at any location. Unanimously, these colleagues stated in such instances that all of their patients exhibited too high measurement values, which could not be decreased in using low frequency current impulses of lowest intensity. In some colleagues, however, I had to realize that when using the technique for decreasing elevated values down to the normal value of 50, they did not take the lowest current intensity thus disregarding the setting between 0–1 in the Diatherapuncteur and between 0–0,1 in the Dermatron.

Another mistake was that when decreasing a maximum value which was reached by a corresponding pressure after the measurement current had established the contact to the points, this pressure was maintained for further therapy. When decreasing is done in using maximal pressure, this constant pressure will damage the point by additional mechanic irritation causing too high and faulty values. After decreasing the point down to 50 and using only minimal pressure for therapy, the doctor in EAV may control his measures by increasing the pressure to realize that there will be no rise of measurement values in sufficient decreasing. Should values yet rise by another 10 scale units, a few further current impulses should be applied.

On this occasion I should like to point to another mistake of the beginner when decreasing. When a point is decreased in using direct current low frequency impulses of least current intensity to result in an increase of the measurement value after applying the first current impulses of least current intensity, this point has not been located properly. Because of the current impulse on an adjacent point close to the measurement point itself, the current has found its own pathway to the measurement point to establish the contact after the first impulse. This is when the correct reading is obtained, or even a possible indicator drop not existing before. Because of the rise of the indicator the beginner tends to believe that the instrument is of no use for decreasing. In this case, the instrument is not to be blamed, but rather the novice himself.

Locally conditioned disturbances.

These may be due to various reasons, mainly, however, to electrical fields of different shapes created by:
1. fluorescent tubes (neontubes), also, by pear-shaped bulbs,
2. cables installed without electric shielding and surrounding the examination place,
3. electric mains hidden in the wall of the examination place,
4. electric instruments not shielded properly.

to 1.:
Fluorescent tubes cause disturbances when not properly grounded. Then, they spread electric fields of up to 1.5 m around the tube. When being measured the patient should keep off a fluorescent lamp by at least 1.5 m with respect to any part of his body. The gratings below such lamps can be grounded (earthed), but the electricians usually fulfil this request only reluctantly. The pear-shaped bulb, in contrast, only builds up an electric field of appr. 0.5 m around itself, causing only occasionally a disturbance.

With respect to the fluorescent neon tube I have to point out that they may be the reason for the daily occurrence of headaches when mounted above the working place. After moving the working place by appr. 1.5 to 2 m away from the fluorescent light, headaches may disappear without the need for taking medications. The same applies to the EAV working place. When it is moved 1 to 2 m aside with respect to the fluorescent light, readings suddenly turn out to be normal. The electric field of a pear-shaped bulb occasionally may irritate a patient, in particular a sensitive one suffering from excitations of the brain stem. The brain stem is the location of the autonomic centers for the circulation and respiration.

In an introductory course held in Stuttgart a colleague doing exercises in EAV reported that at two places where exercises were carried out he could not obtain an indicator drop on the summation measurement point for the arteries (9. Circulation), whereas at a third place he did obtain a drop on this point. I had to confirm these results after reassuring.

At the third working place there existed a distance of 15 cm only to a very low suspended illumination fixture containing a pear-shaped bulb. Thus, the electric field could irritate his brain stem.

to 2.:
Basically speaking, only electrically shielded cables should be used in the vicinity of the examination place. EAV instruments are fitted with these. The EAV instrument should be plugged in a socket which has been grounded (earthed). In one specific case, Dr. *Werner* found out that the socket was connected in a wrong way thus making work impossible for this colleague. The grounding lead was connected to the power lead. This had been done by an apprentice whose work had not been controlled afterwards.

When an EAV instrument cannot be connected to a grounded socket and an elongation lead (cord) has to be used, the connecting coupling should also be shielded and grounded.

to 3:
Vertical and horizontal mains in rooms differ from the main supply cable reaching the electric meter in the house. The electric power may enter the house via the roof from long distance open air power lines or via the basement from underground cables. For taking current from the open air power line, a rack is mounted on the roof of the house. For both forms of current entering the house, reinforced tubing is employed. Since these electric mains from the roof to the basement are only fitted in the staircase in order to avoid living rooms and passing through closets only in very exceptional cases, an influence caused by the mains is practically excluded.

There are, however, exceptions. Thus, I met a female patient who suffered from headaches occurring regularly in the morning also associated with tiredness. The mains in an old house passed behind the bed of this patient. After removing the mains, the headaches in the morning were gone. Mains for distributing the current in the room may irritate unless placed in re-inforced tubes and may cause disturbances in patients. Behind the examination place in EAV there must be no electric lead (cord) when the place is situated next to the wall in order to cancel out a considerable affection of the back of the head, of the nape, and of the back of the patient. To be safe from electric fields caused by leads in the wall, it is best to locate the examination place far away from the wall in the middle of the room.

to 4.:
Electrical instruments not shielded properly are chiefly instruments of old design. They may spread electrical fields thus disturbing the environment. An EAV examination room should not contain such electrical instruments: under no circumstances should there be x-ray instruments, artificial solar light sources, or ozonizing apparatuses which may ionize the air in the room considerably. An ionization makes the air conductive. The electro-stative field collapses. Well tuned short-wave instruments, when started, emit electric alternating fields into the space.

Electrically disturbing fields from adjacent rooms.

These fields may originate in one's own appartment or in the neighbour's appartment in serial houses, also, from the appartment above or below, to interfere with the examination place. One may protect oneself against such disturbing influences intruding from adjacent rooms by attaching metal – or copper foil, or grounded meshed copper – or brass wire to the wall. Wall-paper may be fixed on top of this. Disturbing fields penetrating from below may be kept off by placing a copper sheet under the EAV examination place which should be grounded (earthed). This copper sheet must be covered with a carpet containing no synthetic fibres, with a cocoa mat, a rattan mat, or similar natural tissues. The patient must not be grounded when being examined, since this would lead to faulty measurement results otherwise. A grounding below the examination place protects against terrestrial influences simultaneously.

Electrically distrubing fields from the roof.

Disturbing fields from the roof caused by open air electric lines are very rare. Occasionally, they are present in flat roofs. Rooms under a common gable roof or a double gable roof are most unlikely to be used as medical offices. The kind of the open air power line is also of importance. Normally, four wires are used on the roofs for polyphase current at 220 to 380 volt. Electrical fields caused in West Germany by such wires may be 1–2 m in extension. When there are only two wires (phase and ground) on the roof in older systems, which is an exception to-day, the electrical fields may be up to 5–6 m large. Medical offices close to open air power lines should be rather exceptional. However, open air power lines as often as not build up an electric field around them of 45 to 50 m.

Effects of electrical fields caused by open air power lines in the street.

Overhead wires for street cars (trams) and trolley buses produce fields of permanent magnitudes which may irritate sensitive persons. It is recommended to carry out EAV in a room remote from the street when medical offices are situated close to street car or trolley bus lines. Also, in the immediate vicinity of an electric railway there may be stray currents which may have a disturbing effect on copper plates buried in the soil for grounding (earthing) the rooms of the medical practice. These plates may pick up stray currents to lead them into the house.

Disturbing fields caused by black-and-white TV sets.

High tension transformers of unipolar black-and-white TV sets of the 50s produce disturbing fields which occasionally spread through the wall behind the TV set into the neighbouring room or appartment. Modern black-and-white TV sets no longer exhibit these effects, nor do coloured TV sets to any appreciable amount.

Further disturbing factors in the EAV examination room.

When the floor of the examination room is covered with carpets or carpet patches made of synthetic material, the patient may pick up the electro-static charge from the floor with his bare feet to assemble it on the surface of his body. This may result in a retarded flow of energy in the meridians below the skin in patients suffering from a bad overall energetic situation, that is, energetic blocks in the body and a lack of energy supply in the periphery will result. In these electro-statically charged patients one will find depressed values on the hand and foot measurement points ranging between 50 and 60 without indicator drops (IDs), sometimes even lower. These measurement values, however, are unlikely in view of the patient's complaints. At this level of the values obtained indicator drops will no longer show up. When the floor of the examination room is covered with synthetic material, it should be covered with cotton towels, rattan or cocoa mats made of natural products. Thus, the patient would not pick up electrical charges as he walks to the examination place from the chair where he deposited his clothes.

Factors disturbing the examination due to synthetic material worn on the skin.

Those who want to wear biologic material will never use artificial synthetic products on the skin, but rather prefer cotton under the synthetic material. However, the human body is not equally sensitive to direct skin contacts of synthetic substances on all of its portions. Stockings made of artificial silk worn by female patients do not disturb, nor do hoses. But hip girdles or garters made of synthetic fibres may irritate patients considerably, when their energy production is inconstant or deficient in the first place. But when such patients are charged with low frequency current impulses of a stronger current intensity (tingling), one may notice that this does not succeed. Only after removing the hip girdle the patient can be charged. Why is this so? In acupuncture, the wonder vessel of Tae-Mo is known, also called girdle vessel. This is the only wonder vessel running horizontally in acupuncture. It comprises the whole of the minor pelvis combining all vertical meridians, such as the governor vessel, the conception vessel, the urinary bladder meridian with its two branches, the meridian of the gallbladder, of the spleen-pancreas, of the stomach, of the liver, and of the kidneys. A hip girdle made of synthetic material and being firmly pressed on the skin below the anatomic girdle line, because of pressure and friction, causes a strong electro-static charge which in turn will disturb the energy flow in all of the mentioned meridians and vessels.

What synthetic material, worn on the surface of the body, is capable of doing, I was able to realize in a 64 year old female patient who had been on a cure previously in Bad Orb. She disclosed to me that she had felt worse each day in spite of rest and the execution of the prescribed applications of this cure. My tests taking longer than 3/4 of an hour did not yield any tangible results. The tests just did not make sense. In search of disturbing fields I also thought of synthetic material worn on the skin to find out that the hip girdle was not made of synthetic material. Finally, the patient revealed that she was wearing a wig, whose hairs were attached to a base made of synthetic material.

After removing the wig, I was able to carry out diagnostics and medication testing. This resolved the complaints of the patient, as she had received this wig 8 days before leaving for Bad Orb. Since the wig disturbed her, she was feeling worse each day, in that it disturbed her energetic flow of the vessels and meridians running across the skull, these being governor vessel, urinary bladder meridian, gallbladder meridian, and stomach 1. The energetic passage in these meridians was disturbed by the electro-static charge. In this, it is important to note that the gallbladder meridian traversing the skull by a number of lines contains the measurement points for the midbrain and the interbrain.

The ideal pre-requisites for the EAV examination room and its immediate vicinity.

1. free from powered electro-medical appliances incl. wireless and TV.
2. keep examination place off the wall, which contains electrical leads.
3. no fluorescent neon tubes for lighting purposes. Better lamps as pear-shaped bulbs.
4. a separate room disconnected with adjacent rooms avoiding the transition of ionized air into the examination room.
5. as flooring, wood or linoleum covered with a carpet of natural material e.g., rattan, cork, cocoa mats.
6. the examination chair should be placed on a podium. It should have a lining of natural material to avoid electro-static charges; the feet should be placed on a cotton towel.
7. installation of a large wash basin in the room or in a neighbouring room for bathing the lower arms of patients sweating easily. Such a wash basin for the total length of the lower arm has to be 50x33 cm in its inner dimension.
8. a facility to spray or wash the feet in patients sweating severely.
9. when a new house is built including a medical office, the floor should be grounded (earthed).

Finally, it should be emphasized that in modern hospital buildings, rooms for ECG examinations have to be free from electric fields in order to achieve examination results as precisely as possible. The pre-requisites for a proper examination place in EAV, therefore, are not unusual.

ELECTRO-ACUPUNCTURE
according to Dr. Voll with

EAV – Dermatron or   – Junior
    – Analyzer   – Recording unit
    – Portable unit   (with value and pressure recording)

EAV-DERMATRON with Variopit

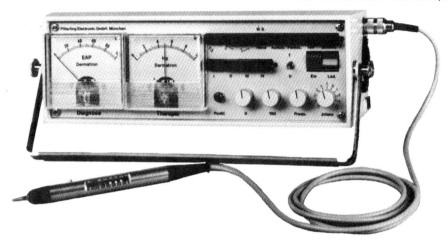

facilitate:
- functional organ and tissue diagnostics via the energy exchange
- therapy with low-frequency relaxation oscillation pulses
- testing of medicine

Portable EAV unit with Variopit

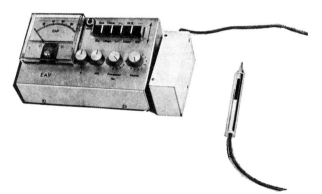

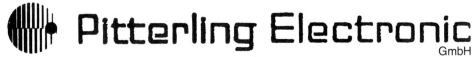

Pitterling Electronic
GmbH

AKADEMIESTRASSE 5, D-8000 MÜNCHEN 40, TELEFON (089) 34 72 81 und 34 70 07